"Rachelle Breslow's book is an inspiring account of one woman's refusal to take on the pessimism of conventional doctors about multiple sclerosis—and of her search for ways to stimulate the healing system of the body/mind. This is a good read."

> — Andrew T. Weil, M.D., author of *Health and Healing* and *Natural Health, Natural Healing*

"*Who Said So?* is the most inspiring book I've read in years. Whether healthy or ill, we all have much to learn about ourselves as we follow Rachelle Breslow's remarkable and courageous journey from a life-threatening illness to enlightenment and health. No one who reads her story can doubt the connection between mind and body."

> — Lillian B. Rubin, Ph.D., clinical psychologist and author of *Worlds of Pain*, *Intimate Strangers*, and *Just Friends*

"Her book is an account not only of her apparent recovery but also—maybe more importantly—of her growth in self-understanding and her increasingly positive attitude . . . Her overarching message is one of hope and the possibility of chan

> — *Booklist*

Who Said So?

Who Said So?

Rachelle Breslow

CELESTIAL ARTS
BERKELEY, CALIFORNIA

Reader, Please Note

The author does not directly or indirectly dispense medical advice or prescribe the use of diet or anything else as a form of treatment for sickness or disease in any form without medical approval.

It is not the intent of the author to diagnose or prescribe. It is the author's intent merely to share experiences and information in order to help you cooperate with your doctor in your mutual quest for health.

In the event that you use the information contained herein without the approval of your doctor, you are prescribing for yourself, which is your right; but the publisher and author assume no responsibility.

Cover design by Ken Scott
Text design by Jeff Brandenburg
Composition by Jeff Brandenburg

FIRST PRINTING, 1991

Library of Congress Cataloging-in-Publication Data

Breslow, Rachelle, 1924–
    Who said so? : a woman's journey of self discovery and triumph over multiple sclerosis / Rachelle Breslow.
        p.   cm.
    Includes bibliographical references (p.).
    ISBN 0-89087-630-4
    1. Breslow, Rachelle, 1924—Health. 2. Multiple sclerosis—Patients—United States—Biography. 3. Multiple sclerosis—Alternative treatment. I. Title.
RC377.B74   1991
362.1'96834'0092—dc20
[B]   90-24623
                                           CIP REV

2   3   4   5   6   7   8   9   0   /   95   94   93

Acknowledgments

With deepest appreciation and love to:

Diana Young—for her unrelenting encouragement, enthusiasm, vision and belief in me and the project.

Lily & Raymond Ayoub—for their unwavering interest, remarkable depth, spirit and loving friendship.

Andrew Weil, M.D.—for his interest and encouragement—and for his validation of my experience in healing from his vantage point of scientific scholarship . . . and for his exceptional books on health, healing and the mind/body connection.

Amritji Desai—for his inspirational message and his gentle influence in my transformation from a human "doing" to a human "being."

Beth Vance—for her inspiration and loving kindness.

Paul, Miriam & Jesse—(my brothers and sister, and their spouses, Gertie, Phil & Ethel) for all their support, fun and love throughout the years.

Steve, Dave & Terri—My three incredible children and their spouses (Margie, Gale & Clay) for their compassion and tolerance during the writing of this book, understanding that I had to look back (with all of its ramifications) in order to go forward.

Andrea, Jessica, Kyle, Max, Melissa & Tripp—my six grandchildren who were a constant source of much cherished renewal by their penetrating sweetness and fun . . . and for their unconditional acceptance and love . . . *the best!*

And to all the incredibly beautiful people at Celestial Arts.

Dedication

To my three loving children, Steve, Dave and Terri, who through the years have helped me to learn the important lessons in life.

I sincerely appreciate each of you for your unique individuality and for all of your many admirable qualities, as I witness how responsibly you are all living out your own realities.

I especially appreciate your ever-present support, kindness, consideration, courage and love . . . and for the pleasure and privilege of being your mother.

Words could never describe the love and gratitude I feel for all of you, so with a full heart I simply say "thank you for all you are to me and for all you have allowed me to be to you."

Contents

All who joy would win must share it
Happiness was born a twin.
—Lord Byron

Terrifying Darkness; Then a Glimmer of Light

*... regular doctors tend to pay attention
only to physical bodies, ignoring the
mental and spiritual aspects of human
beings that are always involved in health
and illness.*

— Dr. Andrew Weil in *Health and Healing:
Understanding Conventional and Alternative
Medicine*

The lovely array of flowers from family and friends was a cheerful reminder that there was life outside this room in Millard Fillmore Hospital in Buffalo, New York. I needed the reminder after several days of being examined and re-examined, talked about as though I were not present, patronized by the uncertain smiles of interns who seemed to be more eager to learn from my predicament than to acknowledge me as a person. I had been mulled over, poked, stabbed, blood-drained and spinal-tapped. Now I was waiting for judgment day. Soon I would learn the answer to so many different questions:

Why was I losing my sense of balance and falling so often?

Why did I stagger in the aisles at the supermarket, drawing she-must-be-stoned stares?

Why did I get dizzy amidst bright lights and noise?

Why did I need two hands to hold a cup?

Why couldn't I squeeze a safety pin hard enough to open it?

Why did I find nothing between my fingers when I knew I had picked up my pen?

Why did my fingers feel tingly, like pins and needles?

Why could I no longer hold my arms up long enough to set my hair?

Why did I have to lean on the counter tops in order to stay upright in the kitchen?

Why did my legs feel stiff and my knees buckle?

Why did my right leg drag?

Why couldn't I lift my toes?

Why did I trip going up the stairs instead of picking up my foot?

Why did I have to sit down so often?

Why did I see two lines running down the center of the road where I used to see one?

Why was I overwhelmed with the need to rest?

Why were there times when I thought that if I had to stand a minute longer, I would pass out?

Why couldn't I dance any more?

Why? Why? Why?

I heard a scurrying of feet and a murmur outside my door. *Is he here already? Oh, God, could that be my doctor? What's he going to tell me?* I was scared stiff of the verdict. I shivered, thinking of all my symptoms. As my doctor walked in, I looked down at my sweaty palms. A crushing fear gripped my whole body.

He said, "Good morning," as he crossed the room. The nurse smiled her hello. He asked how I was. "Just a little nervous," I lied. The walls of the room were closing in. Then I blurted it out: "What do you think is wrong with me?"

Lowering his voice, he began to speak slowly and deliberately. He was patiently trying to explain something about the nerve impulses being blocked or distorted and the deterioration of the myelin sheath. My heart quickened as he continued to describe something totally foreign to me. His tone was serious, but his words were vague and he seemed to be wary of giving me specifics. His uncertainty contrasted with the rigid, authoritative frame beneath his starched white jacket.

Hoping to disguise my fear, I finally said, "Doctor, I have the feeling you're being very gentle about something dreadful. Please be more direct with me. What is your diagnosis?"

"Multiple sclerosis," he said, shifting his position uncomfortably. "There is no cure, and there isn't much either one of us can do about it at this time."

A loud voice in my head began screaming: *Multiple Sclerosis. The Killer of Young Adults. The Crippler of Young Adults. Killer of Young Adults. Killer, Crippler, Killer, Killer, Killer, Killer, Killer, Killer.* Oh, how I felt like screaming at the doctor, at everybody: *Not Me. Not Me. Not Me. Not Me. Not Me.* After what seemed like an eternity, I felt a gentle nudge. My eyes slowly began to focus on the doctor again. *Oh, God, it must be true. Why did I have to ask about a diagnosis?* I managed a half-baked smile and said, "See, you ask a foolish question and you really do get a foolish answer."

The doctor ignored my attempt at humor. He was busy telling me that he would arrange for my discharge from the hospital. Then, in a few days, we would meet in his office for consultation.

I entered this hospital for tests and observation, not for the life sentence that I got. I couldn't wait for the doctor and nurse to stop fussing with my chart and get the hell out of my room so I could fall apart.

No sooner had the door closed behind them than that devastating phrase screamed through my head again: *MULTIPLE SCLEROSIS. KILLER OF YOUNG ADULTS. CRIPPLER OF YOUNG ADULTS.* Why was the memory of those awful words so vivid? I recalled hearing the words during a television appeal for research funds. I knew nothing about the illness at the time, but I was annoyed at the strongly worded appeal. Even the desperate need for money did not seem to justify that kind of damaging statement. I was angry that the writer of the appeal wasn't more sensitive to the victims of the disease and to their families.

Well, so much for then. This is now. And I'm the one here with this crippling, deadly seriously, life-threatening disease. I get your message loud and clear, Mr. Fund-raiser. It really is getting to me, right where I live. You couldn't have made it more potent. I got it, right down in my gut. I believe you. It must be true, or you could not say that multiple sclerosis is a crippler and a killer. My doctor said it was incurable. It's getting through to every part of me. Even my body knows it can't be cured. Oh, God. I hope my body doesn't give in before I do. Oh, dear body, please wait. You're the same body I had before I heard this miserable stuff. Don't get weaker on me now because there's no hope. Don't go limp now. Please, please wait.

Darkness hovered about the corners of the room. Strange shadows moved along the walls. I looked around in horror and disbelief. What was I really doing here on a beautiful, crisp, clear day in October of 1968? Was I dreaming? No. I couldn't be. Here it comes again. I quickly clasped both hands over my ears, but that didn't help. The voice in my head blared on: *Please give to multiple sclerosis, the killer of young adults. Help us fight this incurable disease.*

My shoulders quivered as chills ran through me. My sweaty fingers grabbing the top covers, I slid lower and lower between the sheets. I didn't feel a bit safer. Maybe the hospital bed was making me feel so insignificant, so vulnerable, so helpless and so hopeless. *Geez, my head is killing me. I ache all over.*

I opened my eyes. Everything looked black as my whole world came crashing in on me. *Why me? Why multiple sclerosis. Am I the only one who is facing this nightmare? Incurable, the doctor said. There's nothing he can do for me. Strange, I always thought that doctors could heal anything. Isn't that why they are doctors? Why can't they cure the killer of young adults? To whom do I turn? What do I do?* There was no help anywhere, nobody left but me. *God, I feel awful. Nothing could ever be this bad. Why do I feel worse, so much sicker and weaker than I did before I heard those words, multiple sclerosis? Dear Lord, am I going to die. Dear God, just take me fast. I need some peace.*

I thought about death, but it all seemed hazy. I tried to channel my thoughts, to make some sense. But I knew I was losing it. I prayed through my tears for this nightmare to go away. I could hardly see the chair across the room. My head was reeling as everything became one big blur. I had to surrender completely, to relax my entire body. Finally, I just lay there, limp as a wet rag.

I don't know how long I lay there, or how to explain it, but after a while I felt lifted away. I felt extremely peaceful and knew that something deep and beyond my comprehension was happening. The experience that I had in my lowest moment in that room in Millard Fillmore Hospital gave me the strength and hope to fight the verdict I had just been handed by the medical profession. I have never talked about this experience before. I kept it a secret from everyone, for fear no one would understand. I don't completely understand it myself. But I know that during a particular moment I felt as if my conscious mind separated from my body. I actually saw myself and my body at its very best, completely whole, perfectly formed, strong and healthy. It was the most comfortable, perfectly blissful feeling imaginable. This lovely body felt perfect. I felt as if I were traveling through a very long tunnel. There was a glimmer of bright light far off in the distance. I wanted to keep going toward that radiant energy coming through the other end of the tunnel.

I don't know where the lines are drawn between what is explainable and what isn't. Or if the Twilight Zone really exists. However, at the risk of sounding mystical or even spacey, I know that something changed in me at that moment, that I would never be quite the same again. I felt a new sense of belonging, a kind of connectedness and oneness with the universe. Did the shock of the diagnosis take me to a different level of understanding? Or perhaps a higher self was giving me an opportunity to see what I was supposed to have — wholeness. Was it showing me that I was whole and complete, as I was meant to be, even though I laid there with a partially disabled body? Even now, it is difficult to recapture in words the profound feeling of that moment. I have never again felt anything quite like it. The depth of understanding, the message and the feeling were extremely powerful. Little did I know what an influence this brief glimpse of light and wholeness would be and what a difficult struggle it would be for me to attempt to fulfill this destiny, to fully comprehend my relationship to the world around me and to hold on to the connectedness. There were countless times in the ensuing years that I tried to relive the experience. I never could. Nevertheless, that one experience and the ability to recall it and think about it repeatedly gave me the much-needed strength and courage to plod forward, even against the greatest of odds, in the belief that I was doing the right thing for myself.

A Naive Trust in the Medical Experts

*Nature understands no jesting, she is
always true, always serious, always severe,
she is always right and the errors are
always those of man. She despises the man
incapable of appreciating her — and only
to the apt, the pure, and the true, does she
reveal her secrets.*

— Goethe

Having a name to put to all the symptoms
I had been suffering for at least two years was, in some
ways, a great relief. At least I knew that the overwhelming fatigue I had been feeling was real and there was a
reason for it. At times I had felt so tired and weak that
all I could do was rest. As a forty-four-year-old wife
and mother of three children, running a home and very
active in community affairs, I didn't have time for these
debilitating episodes. I tried to ignore them. Then the
numbness and tingling in the toes of my right foot and
the fingers of my right hand started. I went to see my
family doctor.

His explanation was that I was suffering from some
type of neuritis. He counseled me that I couldn't do
much about it. He didn't seem overly concerned. I went
back to my busy life, determined to ignore my symp-

toms when I could, find temporary relief where I could and generally get on with things.

As new symptoms appeared, I tried to dismiss them. My balance was becoming a problem, and I had to hold on to chairs, countertops and furniture to remain steady. I could no longer hold a cup with one hand. I had to rest before an excursion to the grocery store so that I would not stumble in the aisles. Even then, I shuffled unsteadily and drew quizzical stares from the other shoppers.

It may seem strange to say that, even in this condition, I did not feel that anything was terribly wrong. I was of the generation that did not give in to tiredness, which I thought was the cause of the other types of physical degeneration that were happening to me. Even when my right foot began to drag, and I couldn't lift my toes, and my right hand was so weak that it took me twenty minutes to hook a brassiere, I continued to think that more rest was all I needed.

Two years after I had first gone to my family doctor about my symptoms, I went to his office again, this time for a routine pap smear. When I walked in, I must have been dragging my right leg. The doctor's first words to me were, "I don't like the way you're walking. Get up here on the examining table." *So much for hello*, I thought as he pricked my foot with a pin. He evidently found a problem because he told me that he wanted me to see a neurologist as soon as possible. His tone of voice alarmed me as he explained that he didn't know what was wrong. He selected a neurologist for me to see and even set up the appointment for me.

A few days later, I was in the neurologist's office for what turned out to be preliminary tests. These tests were primarily to discover how I reacted to hot and cold, to pin pricks and to scratching. I felt very little and could not actually differentiate between hot and cold.

As I sat in the neurologist's office, I did feel a strange sense of relief. At least I was no longer ignoring these dreadful symptoms. Even more importantly, someone else recognized my misery and was going to do something about it. It felt so good to be in the right hands at last and to have an authority acknowledge the reality of what was happening to me.

Why didn't I face up to my symptoms sooner? I guess I thought I had to suffer in silence. My family doctor, after all, had said there was nothing to worry about, just a little neuritis. After all, we all have some burden to carry. I simply tuned out, in order to get along as well as I could. Meanwhile, my body continued to get deeper into trouble.

At least now I wouldn't have to apologize for being tired all the time. This tiredness, this utter fatigue was so darn difficult to explain to others. I hardly understood it myself. I even felt ashamed that I couldn't perform in my usual manner.

As the neurologist was finishing up the examination, I tried to get him to tell me what he thought. He was noncommittal. He said that he would like to put me in the hospital for more extensive testing. Before I left his office, he had made arrangements for a room for me at Millard Fillmore.

I went home feeling good that finally someone cared enough to do something about the changes in my body and that the fatigue had a physiological source rather than an attitudinal one. I was filled with hope. In my naivete, I thought I was in the best hands and that a cure was imminent.

It is interesting to recall how I began feeling better as soon as I found that the doctor cared enough to do something about what was happening to me. It never occurred to me to care enough, that the caring had to begin with me. I promised myself that I would never live my life so passively again and that I would trust my feelings enough to take the initiative to be more responsible and to be in more control of my life when necessary.

I went into the hospital looking forward to an end to my miserable problem. Just prior to falling asleep in my hospital bed, I remembered something I had read. It was the epitaph of a hypochondriac: "SEE. I TOLD YOU I WAS SICK."

My first exam in the hospital included tests for walking, squatting and trying to hop. The neurologist also checked my hearing, seeing, swallowing and shrugging of shoulders. He tested my cranial nerves, my reflexes and the strength in my arms, legs and fingers. He gave me sensory tests, asking me whether I could feel light touch, pin pricks, vibrations, hot and cold. He checked my coordination, my memory and my thinking. He gave me a spinal tap, also known as a lumbar puncture. This procedure involves the insertion of a thin needle into the subarachnoid space of the spinal column to withdraw some cerebrospinal fluid for a diagnostic evaluation. There were also some tests involving electrodes applied to my scalp in order to detect any slowing or blocking of nerve impulses.

The morning after the last test was done, I got off my hospital bed to go to the bathroom and my right leg gave way completely, causing me to fall to the floor. This had never happened before. I was always able to hold onto something and get around the room. But this morning, while I was still holding onto the bed, I just crumbled to the floor. Frightened and unable to feel my right leg at all, I crawled to the bathroom and back to bed and rang for the nurse. I asked her what had been done to my leg the day before. She told me that some kind of dye had been injected into it but that I shouldn't worry. I asked to see the doctor as soon as he arrived.

When he came in, I told him about my leg. I said it had never been that weak before and certainly never that useless. I asked whether the test could have affected it. He told me that I had had a common reaction to the dye test. He repeated the nurse's reassurance that there was nothing to be concerned about. The weakness caused by the dye was usually temporary, he said. Then he proceeded to tell me about a patient in England who could not walk for some time after this dye was injected into his leg. Eventually, though, the chap's leg recovered.

I was shocked at how casual he was being. I demanded to know whether the dye test had been absolutely necessary. He said it was the only way he could see what was going on inside the leg. I was livid over the fact that I hadn't been consulted or given a choice about subjecting myself to this risky test. Somehow, I felt it wrong to subject an already weak and ailing leg to such toxic foreign matter. If there was no other way to see the inside, then dammit, the doctors could do without the view. To me, this seemed like guinea pig practice, without permission. They had certainly done enough other tests to come to some conclusion. It was cruel and inhumane to inject a leg with more poison just to satisfy the doctor's curiosity and to assure his diagnosis. If a test is risky, why do it? I can justify taking a risk for a cure, but for a test — outrageous. I hoped my body was not too weak to throw off this poison.

Though I said no more to the doctor, I was left with a bellyful of anger and resentment. This was 1968, a time when one didn't speak up to the deity-of-health-on-earth. Who knows? If I questioned the doctor's approach, I might have been a candidate for the mental ward.

I have since read and heard a great deal about doctor-induced illnesses, caused by tests. Consequently, I will always ask, when a test is suggested, whether the test is necessary in proceeding with a cure or if it will help determine treatment. If the test will not make a difference in the treatment, but is just for information and/or experimental purposes, I will probably refuse the test.

MS: Cause Unknown;
Cure Non-existent

*The doctor of the future will give no
medicine but will interest his patients in
the care of the human frame, in diet, and in
the cause and prevention of disease.*
— *Thomas A. Edison*

Shortly after I left the hospital, with the diagnosis MULTIPLE SCLEROSIS ringing in my ears, I met with the neurologist to learn as much as he could tell me about the disease. The first thing he said was that the cause of the disease was unknown and the cure non-existent. He went on to say that I should be checked every couple of months because multiple sclerosis is a degenerative illness of the central nervous system with varying rates of deterioration in the people who have it. The myelin sheath, which is a roll of fat insulating the nerve fibers of the brain and spinal cord, becomes inflamed and starts to break down in people who have MS. Wherever any part of this sheath has been destroyed, nerve impulses are blocked or distorted and the body cannot respond properly to them. Multiple sclerosis means "many scars." A person's particular disabilities depend upon where the scars are. The messages from the brain are carried through the spinal cord to the other parts of the body in much the same way that electricity for a lamp is carried from the plug in the wall outlet to the switch and light bulb. Just as a tear in the insulating material around an electrical wire can cause a short circuit, the scars on the myelin sheath interfere with messages the brain is trying to send to the rest of the body.

MS is the most common central nervous system disease among young adults in the United States. MS afflicts more women than men, more whites than people of other races and more people born in colder climates both north and south of the Equator. Symptoms usually appear in people between the ages of twenty and forty. It seemed that I had suffered most of the symptoms, which include numbness in the limbs, sporadic weakness, disturbances in the sense of balance, incontinence and problems with vision, dizziness, unsteadiness or tremors in the arms and legs. These symptoms appear unpredictably and may disappear without recurrence. The variation in symptoms makes the disease difficult to investigate and understand.

The neurologist did not look at me with pity as he declared how little either of us could do about my condition. He was calm and straightforward, with just a hint of coolness and impatience, which I suspected had something to do with his own frustration at being so limited in what he could offer me. I wondered how many times he had to go through this explanation with other patients and what it felt like to have to admit that he could do nothing.

He could give me cortisone if I wanted it, he said. Remembering the injection of dye into my ailing leg, I interrupted to ask him what cortisone would do against the disease. He said that it was no cure but that it might make me feel better. I got a flash about not needing any more poison to make me feel better if it had nothing to do with a cure. And I decided to refuse cortisone.

The doctor continued his bleak description of MS. He told me I could expect a progressive breakdown of the bodily functions. He said fatigue was a big part of the disease and cautioned me to rest often and not get overtired. When I asked about exercise, he recommended against it because of the fatigue factor. This surprised me. A ditty, popular at the time because of exercise guru Jack LaLanne's use of it, ran through my mind: *Use it or lose it.* Since I was blessed with some movable parts, I wanted to do what I could to keep them moving. I made a mental note to look into different forms of exercise on my own. I knew any further questioning of my doctor would be unproductive. His manner told me just how opposed he was to my trying to figure out an exercise routine or do anything else on my own.

I asked him if there were any foods I should avoid and about diet in general. He crisply informed me that nutrition had absolutely no bearing on MS. He began talking again about the deterioration of the myelin sheath and the mystery surrounding its cause. "When the cause can be determined," he said, "we will be on our way to finding a cure."

I was beginning to get the message. At the time, neither one of us realized how much a part hope plays in a person's healing process. "So, doctor, you're saying that there is nothing I can do to help myself?" I asked quietly.

"Not at this point," he said, getting up from his chair and leaning over his neat, shiny desk. I knew that this was his not-so-subtle way of saying that our consultation was at an end. "Just try not to tire yourself too much and rest often. And make an appointment to see me in about two months, if not sooner." He added what

I'm sure seemed to him like words of hope: "There may be a possible breakthrough to a cure in about five to ten years."

I never saw that neurologist again. I can only hope that the scientific community has progressed to the understanding that there can be many avenues to regeneration and healing.

Retreating Into Secrecy
And Silence

*There's no such thing as false hope. There
is only false no-hope. You cannot tell the
future of an individual. Doctors keep
killing people with their words when they
say there is no hope. Part of why I wrote
another book was to say: The message is to
heal your life, not cure your disease.*
— Dr. *Bernie Siegel in* Love, Medicine
and Miracles

Since that dreary day when I went numb
with apprehension and confusion upon hearing the
prognosis for my disease, I have heard many times that
the patient always seems to take a turn for the worse
when she is told of a hopeless situation. That certainly
was true with me. All of the possible symptoms associated with MS seemed to hit me at once, full force. All I
wanted to do was lie in bed forever. The demands of
my active family, however, made that impossible. I had
three children, ages twenty, sixteen and thirteen. One
of my biggest fears at that time was having them find
out that I had a dreaded killer disease. I simply couldn't
deal with constantly having to bolster their hopes and
relieve their fears when I was desperate for a way to
fortify my own hope and banish my own fears. I think I

knew instinctively that I needed time and energy for thinking through what my own response was going to be to the diagnosis; I felt that too much of the energy I needed would be depleted in dealing with the responses of my children and that I would have nothing left for exploring ways of bettering my situation. I decided to keep the diagnosis a secret from my two sons, Steve and David, and my daughter, Terri. I often felt like a zombie, sleepwalking through chores in order to maintain some semblance of normalcy, to pretend that life in the family could go on as usual. The children were busy with school, work, tennis and various other activities. They did notice my symptoms at one time or another, but I always offered some vague excuse. The one I used most often was that I was just tired and needed more rest. My tone made it obvious that I considered any mention of my symptoms annoying and stressful. I never let them see me use the walker that I eventually acquired to help me move through the house during the day. Only rarely did I rely on a cane in front of them. My children kept busy with their lives, and I avoided any discussion of what might be bothering me.

I kept my diagnosis a secret from friends and acquaintances, too. All I knew was that the fewer people who knew of my situation, the less chance news of it had of reaching my children. I dropped all my community activities. I began to make excuses when social invitations came our way. I invented reasons for skipping the customary visits to the in-laws and to my own relatives, all of whom lived out of state.

I think now that my decision to keep my diagnosis a secret was my way of trying to keep some control over my own life. I knew there was no one I could depend on in the medical community for help. I had only myself. I had to find the strength from within somehow, and I couldn't afford the possibly contagious attitude from others that might foster dependence or self-pity. I knew that it would be difficult to focus on finding ways to improve my health if I permitted others to challenge my decisions. I couldn't afford their well-intentioned concerns or their questions, since I had no logical answers.

I did tell my husband that I had multiple sclerosis. The diagnosis was extremely difficult for him to take. His primary interest in life had always been his work, and he was accustomed to my complete support for all of his concerns and endeavors. He counted on having as his wife a strong woman who didn't show much vulnerability. I tried to keep our marriage as status quo as possible. I made a concerted effort not to talk about my symptoms or MS, and he evidently didn't feel the need or desire to inquire. In retrospect, I think that my willing silence was also motivated by a deep fear that he would abandon me if I couldn't continue to fulfill his needs. His attitude must have triggered some fear of abandonment that I had suffered as a child. This became clearer to me with the passing of time.

At first, however, the pressure of keeping my diagnosis secret from almost everyone and of not being able to talk about it with the one person who was aware of it made my life hell. By day, I held back all of my feelings, repressing and censoring constantly. At night, the unexorcised feelings came back to haunt me. All the fear, panic, depression and exhaustion hit me with brutal force. I couldn't sleep. The clock became my enemy as my eyes would wander to those numbers and I would wish they would tell me it was daybreak so I could busy my mind again with holding the family together. I wanted any distraction from thoughts about my hopeless situation. I don't know how many sleepless nights I spent; I soon lost count.

MS seemed to assert itself in proportion to how much I denied its existence. I began to lose my balance more frequently. My vision blurred, and my hands and fingers became weaker and weaker. I didn't feel slight burns or small kitchen cuts on my fingers. I began to realize that I had to try something on my own, anything to kindle the feeling of hope, to keep from giving in and withering away just waiting for science to find the cure. As I began to listen more and more to my intuition, I realized how little recognition I had given to my own needs, how much I had been living other people's lives and needs while neglecting my own. It had always been so much more important to please others than to please myself. In fact, it was downright mandatory to my well-being that I be needed by others. I had to live for others, no matter what the cost to myself. It took a life-threatening, catastrophic illness to force me to be attentive to my own needs, to go within and to listen to what I was all about.

Breaking Through the
Wall of Hopelessness

*Your body contains all the answers it needs
to keep itself healthy. By getting in touch
with your inner self and by learning to
read the messages of your body, you can
learn things about healing which high-
budget, highly specialized medical research
programs may never discover.*

— Dr. *Mike Samuels in* The Well Body
Book

I spent the next year doing research into all the known methods of healing. I attended health lectures and conventions. I read all the latest medical journals and the literature in the medical school libraries. I browsed the books in the health food stores. I spoke with many who had helped themselves to better health. Gradually, I began to put into practice whatever made sense to me. I insisted that whatever I added to my health-care regimen be chemical-free, non-toxic and safe, posing absolutely no risk to my body and/or health. Beyond those restrictions, I wanted to remain open to every possibility.

During this time of casting about for ways to treat myself, I visited the local chapter of the Multiple Sclerosis Society. I was not seeing any kind of physician, and

I felt the need for contact with professionals familiar with the disease. I wanted to find out if there was anything new I could possibly do for myself. I almost didn't keep my appointment because I became so discouraged while I was waiting in the reception area for the nurse to take my history. The room was filled with people in wheelchairs; they appeared to be so defeated by life that I wanted to turn and run. Seeing my future staring back at me was too much. I steadied myself and kept my place. The nurse finally came to get me. She asked me to become part of a long-term research project, which meant that I would have to return to the office once a month to have blood samples taken. I agreed. As I continued to return to the place where defeat was so palpably in the atmosphere, my own condition deteriorated. After several visits, I left the society's office with a three-footed cane to help me walk. Soon that cane was not sturdy enough to support me. My balance was becoming more of a problem, and I was falling more often. I had to turn my cane in for a walker. This was one of the saddest days of my life. I felt more desperate than ever.

Shortly after I got my walker, I was reading the newspaper when an article on acupuncture caught my eye. A little light flashed inside my head, and I knew I had to follow my instinct to try this. There was no acupuncturist in Buffalo at that time. Through some digging and several contacts, I made an appointment with an acupuncturist associated with St. Luke's Hospital in New York City. Dr. Shyh-Jong Yue gave me eight treatments over the course of one month. During the first treatment, he placed more than ten very thin needles into my wrists, feet and back. I felt absolutely no pain and lost not a drop of blood; the needles left no holes or scars. At the end of a month of treatments, I was able to walk, unaided, down the long corridor, into the elevator and out to the car, which was parked two blocks away. Fantastic! It had been well over three years since I could walk that far without having to stop to rest along the way. I was elated.

Dr. Yue told me before I left that my new-found strength, energy and nerve stimulation might not last with so few acupuncture sessions. He was right. My renewed strength and mobility lasted only a short time. But that did not make one bit of difference to me. I was so ecstatically happy to learn that my body parts had not atrophied and were not dying before me. I was totally enveloped with anticipation and hope. For the first time, I knew that some improvement was possible, that there were ways I could make a difference in my own body and health. The resolve and determination I had after those acupuncture sessions were indescribable.

Acupuncture was a breakthrough experience for me even though it was by no means a cure. I was not concerned with cures. I was just so excited for any improvement, for any indication of potential for further improvement. Dr. Yue's eight acupuncture treatments taught me a tremendous life-enhancing lesson about how my miraculous body works and how important it is too keep an open mind and to seek possibilities, no matter what the authorities and the experts say. The treatments taught me that I am more responsible for my health and well-being than anyone else and that I have to have the confidence to trust my own intuition and ability to follow through with what is best for me. I began to appreciate the resourcefulness that we all have at our disposal. And I marveled at my body's natural recuperative powers. Rejuvenation was possible. There was hope!

The doctors, at that time, thought that the deterioration of the myelin sheath was permanent; so they did not look into repair. My own acupuncture treatments proved to me that the degenerative process was not irreversible. If the needles that were placed on the meridian points made contact and stimulated energy to flow once again, I felt assured that there was still life in that area. Even if the improvement was temporary, it encouraged me and gave me confidence that I was on the right track. What an incredible difference that made.

When the physical improvements from treatment wore off, none of the mental improvements did. I knew that the insights acupuncture had given me were only the beginning. I had much work left to do. I felt such hope. And I found myself starting to ask, *Who said so? Who said this disease could only go downhill? Who said it had to get worse? Who said that I shouldn't exercise? Who said that diet didn't matter? Who said that nothing could be done until a cure was found? Who said so? Who said so? Who said so?*

How do they know if they've tried for a cure only in the laboratory? How do they know if they are looking for a drug or a surgical cure? How much do they know about how to enhance healing naturally? How much do they know about the powers of the body to heal and rejuvenate itself? How much do they look into, above and beyond the medical curriculum at medical school?

However much they knew, doctors had nothing to offer me. I knew that I needed to search on my own, that there was no authority who would agree with me or even encourage me to seek elsewhere. As long as I listened to them, I had no hope. As long as I listened to the traditional medical professionals, I would remain a victim of the "killer of young adults, the crippler of young adults." That miserable, impossible phrase had hypnotized me with fear. My doctor's authoritative opinion had sent me to a deeper level of immobility. I was stunned to realize how much the belief that my situation was hopeless had affected the way I felt physically. I was stunned to realize how a negative prognosis had blocked any other possibilities or any creative thinking. When acupuncture revealed to me that my body could still respond and recuperate, I felt all the systems in my body begin to signal go again. My new-found motivation, resolve and hope knocked me off the complacency trip. There are no words to describe the 180-degree turn in my attitude. I felt the endorphins in my brain giving birth all over the place. Exhilarating!

I knew my search would not be easy. I knew that there was no authority who would agree with me or even encourage me. I knew I still had all the original symptoms. But I was also aware that I had a choice in what I believed. I was aware of all the stuff out there in the world coming at us daily. I realized that what we choose to buy into affects us in ways that go deep into our bodies. The realization was astounding, becoming clearer and clearer. If what I believe about what I'm told can so effectively impress me into negative belief, blocking any further possibility, and that belief can manifest itself in some physical way — then why can't the reverse also be true? It must be true. That's exactly what was happening. As soon as I found some good reason to be hopeful and motivated, my belief turned to a positive one, which obviously had a positive effect on me physically. It must be just how the placebo works.

Aha. What a discovery. Just maybe if I can consciously try to monitor my thoughts and beliefs and accept only the positive messages, if I can influence my mind to be impressed only with positives, then my body may not have to work so hard to overcome all that negative garbage manifesting there, all that holds me back from seeing the possibilities.

I can only speculate about where I would be now had I looked at the negative rather than the positive aspect of my acupuncture experience. I might have wailed, "Oh, God, the acupuncture didn't last. It didn't work. Nothing will ever work. The doctors were right. I can only sit around and wait for their cure, while I'm miserable and degenerating. I should have taken their advice and saved my energy and not gotten my hopes up." And surely, their prognosis would have come true.

Instead, I took the positive side of the experience. The positive attitude that helped me twenty years ago has since been validated by such figures as Norman Cousins, Dr. O. Carl Simonton, Dr. Andrew Weil and Dr. Bernard Siegel. By taking the positive side of the acupuncture experience to heart, I had the courage to continue trying other things on my own. I believed in hope and in the miracles of rejuvenation and recuperation. It is incredibly impressive to me that because of the positive reinforcement of the acupuncture experience, I felt a whole new belief system taking hold in my mind. All my systems were in open, positive alignment for healing and success. I had the momentum now.

When the Student Is Ready, the Teacher Will Appear

> *The only prerequisite for learning to take responsibility for one's health is to discard concepts that stand in the way and adopt more useful ones. It is not just scientists who benefit from new conceptual models. Anyone who comes to see healing as an innate capacity of the body rather than something to be sought outside it, will gain greater power over the fluctuations of health and illness. Anyone who recognizes the importance of mind and belief in determining responses to treatments will be able to make better sense of past interactions with medical practitioners and better decisions about future ones.*
>
> — *Dr. Andrew Weil in* Health and Healing: Understanding Conventional and Alternative Medicine

I absolutely cannot emphasize enough the importance and the value of belief and its positive or negative effect on human physiology, especially down at the cellular level. Since doctors are trained to believe that once the myelin sheath is damaged, it cannot be repaired, they do not try to find ways of repairing it. Because I refused to believe in the irreversibility of my losses, my body was able to set about building a new set of sheaths and restoring function to its nerves. At every hurdle in the healing process, I would ask myself, *Who said so?* My byword bible became: *While seeing is believing, experiencing is truth.* Until I experienced something, it was not true for me. In this context, I learned that there is no such thing as incurable, that when a doctor says something is incurable, he really (and more accurately) is saying that the medical community has not yet found a cure. Who can accurately predict anything? The facts are never in. Saying that a disease is incurable and saying that a cure has not been found are two entirely different statements.

Near the end of 1969, I read in the *Buffalo Courier Express* that a Dr. Roy L. Swank, professor of neurology at the University of Oregon Medical School, was going to be speaking in our city. He reportedly had vast experience with multiple sclerosis patients. I attended his lecture and heard about a special low-fat diet that had helped his patients who started the diet in the earlier stages of the disease. He referred to the Far Eastern countries where there was virtually no MS among the population and attributed this to the heavy rice and low-fat diets prevalent in those countries. After the lecture, I asked Dr. Swank if he had heard about the rice diet being used for a variety of health problems by a Dr. Kempner at Duke University in Durham, North Carolina. He said he had heard of the diet and that it was more stringent than the one he used but would be a good place for me to start. The next day, I called Duke University to find out what I could about the rice diet.

The program at Duke required at least a four-month commitment. My youngest child was fourteen. I thought I could leave the family for four months. I got the family together and told everyone about the program and why I thought it would help me. I still had not told them of my diagnosis. They knew something was wrong because of my chronic fatigue. When I asked for their cooperation, they were unreservedly enthusiastic about my going and immediately began to talk about who would be responsible for what at home in my absence. They were also, all during my journey back to health, unanimous that the family income should support whatever steps I felt I had to take for my recovery.

For a long time, I had harbored a feeling of being nutritionally out of balance. However, if I attempted to discuss this with doctors, I was told that nutritional changes were nonsense. Dr. Walter Kempner, however, had different ideas about the importance of diet. His tests showed that I did suffer some nutritional deficiencies. I was his only MS patient at the time. Others in my group were suffering from various problems, including heart disease, nephritis, ulcers, cancer, obesity, hypertension and diabetes. While I was on the rice diet, I did feel better. Some strength returned to my fingers and leg. However, I returned home earlier than intended since the diet was too stringent for me to remain on the full four months. I planned to adapt some of what I had learned to my own nutritional practices.

About this time, I also began a program of moving and stretching. I laid on the floor for support. Because of my weakness and poor balance, I was not able to do much. But I was determined to move anything that could still move and to keep at it every day regardless of the results. My fingers and toes were too weak to move on their own so I would sit on the floor and turn each finger and toe manually, up and down and around. When I learned that water assumes about ninety percent of body weight, I decided that a pool would be the best place for me to exercise. I could move much more easily in water. I went to the pool almost every day and got good results from those sessions.

At this point, it occurred to me that I was very slowly improving despite having been told there was no cure for MS. Was it possible that I did not actually have MS after all? Maybe I had been misdiagnosed and should seek another medical opinion. I wound up going to five different neurologists and other medical specialists. All these practitioners told me essentially the same thing: "You have multiple sclerosis, and it is incurable. There is nothing we can do about it at this time. There is nothing you can do about it either, so try to live with it in the very best way that you can."

I automatically translated their words to fit my new belief system. What I heard them say was: *We think MS is incurable since we have not been able to come up with a drug and/or surgery that will correct or cure it. But that doesn't mean that you yourself cannot do something about it. Go home, experiment, be your own expert.* I actually came away from those visits feeling good since I was proving that I could make a difference in my own condition by taking control and following my own instincts. I was becoming my own best authority on myself and on my own body and health. Perhaps this is how all kinds of discoveries are made.

Nothing of worth ever runs smoothly, especially where learning and progress are concerned. I felt terribly frustrated and confused much of the time in those early years. There was so much contradiction in the information I read. I had no authority to consult. No medical professional would even consider discussing alternatives or any treatment of a non-medical nature. I tried to remain open to anything that wasn't risky to my health. But at times I wondered, *What do I do now?* The problem was downright overwhelming. I had a running argument in my head between the doctors telling me not to waste my precious energy on such foolish pursuits and my inner self telling me that defeat comes to no woman until she admits it to herself. I thought I had more to learn, but often I did not know which direction to turn.

I began talking to myself, giving myself pep talks. These became habitual and went something like this: *Okay, Rach. Settle down and try to think this through. First of all, always remember the acupuncture experience, which taught you that movement and improvement in your body are always possible. Don't be too concerned about the lack of total agreement over any method. Remember how critical and unbelieving the doctors were about acupuncture. Some even called this 5,000-year-old treatment "quack-upuncture." Yet you, dear Rach, were open enough to try it. It worked for you. It proved to be invaluable. So feel confident that you can sort all of this out and something will turn up. If you wait until you see the next step with perfect clarity, you will never do anything. Maybe you're not supposed to know what lies ahead. Any fool can count the seeds in one apple, but only the highest power can count the apples in one seed. So trust in the process and go for it. Just relax and listen to your intuition and start anywhere again. You'll know what to do when the time is right. When the student is ready, the teacher will appear. Be ready. Stay open.*

A mental image that I often used for comfort was of the time I was driving alone in a blizzard. I was trying not to panic even though I could not see anything through the blanket of snow. I couldn't stop because of the cars behind me. But I could see the back of the car in front of me. Just being able to see the lights of that one car ahead got me safely to my own driveway. I had no choice but to follow what I could see and move one car-length at a time home.

I made a commitment to myself to stay open and to take inspiration where I could find it. One of the public figures who helped me most at that time was the actress Patricia Neal. Whenever I felt frustrated or impatient about my rate of progress, I remembered the story of her struggle back to health. Two years after winning an Academy Award for her performance in *Hud* (in 1963), she suffered a series of massive strokes. She was confined to a wheelchair, and her speech was severely impaired. Through extensive physical therapy, tender loving care and her own belief that she would get better, she did recover; she returned to the screen in 1968. Her courage, tenacity, faith and hope inspired millions of people. I was definitely one of them.

Another person who helped me a great deal was the nutritionist Adelle Davis. In her book *Let's Get Well,* she discussed multiple sclerosis, reporting that autopsies of MS victims had shown a marked decrease in the lecithin content of the brain and the myelin sheath. Both of these areas are normally high in lecithin. In MS sufferers, however, not only is the lecithin content abnormally low but what lecithin there is in the brain and the myelin sheath is abnormal, containing saturated, instead of unsaturated fatty acids. Davis recommended adding three or more tablespoons of lecithin to the daily diet of people with MS; those who followed her recommendation showed great improvement, she claimed.

Adelle Davis was a biochemist who believed that there was much evidence to show that most degenerative diseases are caused by deficiencies in diet and allergies to poisons used as preservatives, sprays and additives in our food. Her work with the autopsies of MS victims intrigued me. I read everything else I could find about lecithin and attempted to work out a nutritional program following the advice in her books.

When I thought I had a workable food and supplement plan, I contacted Davis through a mutual friend. I sent her a detailed copy of my plan, which consisted of a diet of raw vegetables, fruit, grains and raw nuts, plus the supplements I thought I needed. I hoped I had gotten the right balance. Supplements were especially tricky because one might deplete others if not combined correctly. I had dropped all meat, fish, fowl and store-bought baked goods from my diet. I avoided foods with additives, preservatives and saturated fats. Davis wrote back to me, commending me on the plan I had put together. "You have done a good job on your own," she said, in the first line of her letter. You can imagine the high I felt reading that line. Wow. Here was a real, live authority telling me that I was on the right track. After nearly three years of seeking and searching blindly to help myself, to do whatever I could to get a handle on this dreadful disease, here was an expert telling me I was doing a good job. The positive reinforcement was great. I will always remember her for the feeling of hope and support she gave me.

A couple of months after she wrote to me, Davis came to Buffalo to give a talk to the medical students at the University of Buffalo. She said she would like to meet me and asked me to spend some time with her after her lecture. I jumped at the opportunity. I remember being so impressed by the way the president of the third-year medical students introduced her. He said: "Fellow students, up to now we have learned a great deal about disease. Tonight we are going to learn something about health."

I think Adelle Davis was instrumental in bringing the whole idea of prevention to the attention of the medical community at the same time as she was educating the public. I am very grateful to her and others like her who took a lot of flack in their attempts to enlighten the consumer and who tried to make all the doctors of the world more like people and all the people of the world more like doctors. I am grateful for the times I got to spend with her. Unfortunately, she was suffering from cancer when I met her. She had been given heavy doses of radiation as a child for a bone ailment. I had only a few times with her after our initial meeting.

Noticeable Progress

By this time in my self-treatment, three years after MS was diagnosed, I was making noticeable progress. I was on my vegetarian diet, with no meat fish or fowl. And I was doing stretching exercises in a swimming pool on a consistent basis. My physical stamina was much improved. I could now make a reasonable fist, curl my toes, rotate my ankles, walk farther, hold a needle and sew and work for longer and longer periods of time. Those daily practices that we all take for granted but that had been denied me for so long were coming back within my grasp. However, I still had to rest often. I still felt some weakness in my right hand and leg. I still had some dizziness and poor balance at times.

I began looking for other kinds of self-treatment. At the local spa where I went for my water exercises, one of the instructors suggested that I try a body massage. He said that would make me less stiff and give my muscles some much-needed relaxation. That sounded wonderful to me. I knew that to balance myself at times I was putting stress and pressure on the stronger parts of my body. I had never considered massage as a way to relieve the kind of body tension that such compensation caused. The super deep massage therapist to whom I went did wonders for me. The parts of my body that I was using to compensate for the weaker parts were forever grateful for the incredible relief and release that massage gave them. Massage had other benefits as well: It compensated for lack of exercise in restricted areas. It heightened tissue metabolism and increased tissue nutrition. It increased the secretion of fluids and waste products via the kidneys. And it encouraged nitrogen, phosphorous and sulphur retention for bone repair.

The massage therapist also did some reflexology on my feet. Reflexology, also called acupressure, zone therapy or shiatsu, primarily works on nerve endings that correspond to organs and other parts of the body. The therapist taught me to practice reflexology on myself. The idea was to break up any calcification that might interrupt the flow of energy and circulation in the body.

Another tool that I found useful at this time was the slant board. If I laid on it with my head at the bottom and my feet in the air, I could relieve some of the chronic fatigue that I felt. I could feel the effects of gravity reversing themselves.

I was definitely making progress.

Affirmation From a Renegade M.D. in Germany

One Monday morning I was sitting on the floor, doing reflexology on my feet, when my daughter came in with the mail. She gave me the *Organic Consumer Report*, a newsletter published by Betty Morales from Eden Ranch. The headline on the lead article read: "MULTIPLE SCLEROSIS INCURABLE IN U.S. — CURABLE IN EUROPE. WHY?" I couldn't read the article fast enough. My excitement grew as I read the report about a Dr. Joseph Evers, who had been treating MS patients at his clinic in Arnsberg, West Germany, for more than twenty years. Dr. Evers had seen more than 13,000 patients. He had compiled case histories on each one of them. One hundred of his patients, whom he had monitored monthly for twenty years, he considered cured.

I couldn't believe my eyes. Here in black and white, for the very first time, I read that multiple sclerosis was curable. Incredible. A medical doctor had actually kept records to verify this. The most unbelievable part of the whole thing was that it was being completely ignored in the good old United States — no interest whatsoever. I was both angry and elated. The report talked about how Dr. Evers, a fully accredited, licensed medical doctor, had been rejected by his own profession and treated little better than a quack. Meanwhile, MS was on the increase. The medical monopoly was not coming up with any answers and refused to spend a penny of millions of research dollars on the investigation of nutrition or any other lifestyle condition that might affect MS.

I knew I had to find out more about Dr. Evers. Here was yet another sign that countless doors out there were waiting to be opened. *Yeah, right on, Rach. Seek and ye shall find.* I had a dear friend who happened to live about an hour's drive from Dr. Evers's clinic in Germany. I contacted Helga, and she made an appointment for me at the clinic. It was December of 1971 when I met Dr. Evers and spent several hours at his clinic. I was pleasantly surprised to learn that through my own searching I had designed almost exactly the same program that he prescribed for his patients. There was no need for me to stay at the clinic since I was doing so well on my own. I did learn from him about sprouting wheat, and I collected some informational literature.

A typical day at the clinic went as follows:

7:00 a.m.	cool shower, limited to one minute
7:05	swim or water exercises
8:15	exercises
9:15	breakfast
10:00	swim
12:15 p.m.	lunch
1:00	rest
3:00	massage
4:00	stretching exercises
5:00	walk outdoors
5:30	dinner
7:30	massage, then an hour of rest
10:30	bedtime

The visit to the West German clinic gave me more validation and reinforced my belief that I was doing what I needed to do to heal myself, even though the process was painfully slow. When I returned to Buffalo from Germany, I continued with my program of good nutrition, vegetarianism and exercise. I also remained open to other healing methods.

A Trip to Shangri-La

In the winter of 1973–74, my husband had to be away on business for a couple of months. My oldest son was working out of town, and the other two kids were away at college. I was uncomfortable at the thought of being on my own and at the mercy of the icy, snowy Buffalo winter. I was reading a magazine called *Let's Live* when I noticed an advertisement for the Shangri-La Health Resort in Bonita Springs, Florida. My eyes were drawn to the phrase, "Where Health Is Taught." *Wow, could this be true? Is there a place that actually teaches health as a preventive measure?* I was on the phone almost immediately, talking with Dr. R.J. Cheatham, owner/director of Shangri-La. My hope was to do some bartering in exchange for a two- to three-month stay at the warm, healthful resort. We negotiated a four-month stay in exchange for my writing articles, interviewing guests for documentation and doing some promotional and counseling work. I arrived at Shangri-La in December of 1973.

I felt an immediate bond with Dr. Cheatham. We had both gone through a number of similar, difficult experiences in our attempts at healing. He had healed himself of cancer through studying and practicing the principles of natural hygiene. Before he discovered natural hygiene, he had the entire surface of the right side of his chest removed, leaving the bones covered with only a little skin and a scar seventeen inches long. His doctors told him that he could expect to live five years at the most after such an operation. When I met him, it had been twenty-five years since his chest surgery.

Dr. Cheatham had attended a lecture on natural hygiene shortly after his operation. The principles of the laws of nature and their simplicity, logic and common sense impressed him to the extent that he felt he had learned the answer to health and disease, to living and dying. He wholeheartedly embraced the natural hygiene philosophy that disease is not a chance thing; it is the result of definite causes. To have good health, we must eliminate the causes of poor health. He began to practice natural hygiene by, first, going on a detoxifying fast and then by exercising daily, correcting his diet, getting plenty of rest, sun and fresh air and taking daily baths. His physical condition improved dramatically. He had no further recurrences of cancer. He also found that his eyesight improved to the point where he no longer needed the glasses that he had worn for ten years.

Dr. Cheatham suggested that I try the natural hygiene way to health, and I happily agreed. He suggested that I begin by fasting on distilled water only for at least thirty days. I was skeptical about the benefits of this, but I agreed. In my own mind, I thought I would fast for a couple of days and then get on with the business of why I was at Shangri-La. To my amazement, I remained on the distilled water fast for twenty-eight days. I had very little discomfort. So many things were going on at Shangri-La (lectures, work, classes, visits with people from all over the world) that I did not miss food at all.

No one should ever undertake a fast without a doctor's approval and without proper supervision.

Under the right conditions, a fast can be marvelously beneficial. I read Arnold De Vries's book, *Therapeutic Fasting*, while I was at Shangri-La. In it, he writes:

> *Fasting affords the organs of the body the closest possible approach to a complete physiological rest. Many organs are overworked and overstimulated, and hence weakened, through the constant use of defective foods and excessive quantities of foods. During a fast, the necessary work done by the organs is reduced to the lowest possible minimum. As there is no further intake of food, assimilation in the body only involves the redistribution of the elements already stored there. Thus the organs are given a chance to recuperate and restore their vital powers. Repair of damaged structures may take place and the body undergoes a general healing process.*

I broke my fast on the twenty-ninth day with a half glass of freshly juiced grapes, diluted with distilled water. I had never before nor have I since tasted anything quite that delicious. For several days after that, I had a vegetable or freshly squeezed fruit juice at each meal. Then I had fresh fruit for breakfast, fresh vegetable salads and nuts (in the shell) or seeds for lunch and raw vegetables plus one or two cooked vegetables for dinner. This diet made me feel stronger than I ever had. I noticed improvement in every area of my body. I was able to hold myself more erect, to do more and more of the stretching and to walk farther without tiring and without aid. My elimination was better. My hair and skin were healthier looking. I had much less fatigue.

The principles of natural hygiene call for a diet that is approximately eighty percent raw foods. Raw food is live food that will nourish cells, just as seeds grow when planted in the soil. If cooked food is planted, it will not grow; it will lay there and putrefy. When we eat too much cooked food and not enough raw food, with its natural enzymatic action to ensure regeneration and maintenance, putrefaction occurs in our bodies.

When I returned home from Shangri-La, I continued the eating habits I had learned there. My diet was primarily raw foods, and I was careful about the way I combined foods. One food per meal was the ideal at Shangri-La, but for those who wanted a combination of foods the Shangri-La Natural Hygiene Institute published a chart showing which foods could be healthfully combined. (See the chart included in the appendix). I followed the recommendations on the chart. I dropped most of the supplements I had been taking. And I continued to exercise everything that would move. I was slowly getting results.

J'ai Bhagwan

For years I had been intrigued by the notion of learning yoga. Buffalo, however, was not home to any yoga instructors. I made periodic calls to the University of Buffalo in hopes of finding a medical student from India who might consider teaching yoga. But I found no one. I tried to learn some of the postures from books, but I had trouble because of my special problems with balance and movement. Once I was back home from Shangri-La, the desire to learn yoga was persistently in my mind. I made another call to the university medical school, and this time I found someone to get me started. This doctor from India got me started all right, started on a journey that could never have happened any other way, a journey that had far-reaching consequences, a journey that no one could possibly take for me, a journey of a lifetime, a journey within.

The doctor from India told me there was only one yoga teacher or guru that he could recommend to me. The only problem was that the teacher did not live in Buffalo. This was the problem that had kept me from learning yoga before. For some reason, however, distance no longer mattered to me in my quest for health and growth. I told the doctor from India that I was desperate to get in touch with the teacher he knew. He said, "I know you are." There was a mysterious wisdom in his voice that gave me a chill. Then he told me the teacher's name: Yogi Amrit Desai of Sumneytown, Pennsylvania, near Philadelphia.

In 1974, I traveled to the Sumneytown community that Amrit Desai had established. Amrit Desai had been in the U.S. since 1960, when he arrived from India to study fabric design at the Philadelphia College of Arts. From the beginning of his stay in this country, he taught yoga part-time. A demonstration of the postures or asanas that he presented at the International Festival in 1960 gained him such renown that he received many requests from television producers and organizations to give seminars and yoga classes. He believed that the yogic approach to a healthy, happy and centered life could be well-integrated with Western ways. And he devised a method for teaching yoga that could be readily understood and practically applied by Westerners. Eventually, he established an ashram in the peaceful rural community of Sumneytown. The ashram would attract thousands of men and women seeking to realize their potential for personal growth and would be re-named the Kripalu Center for Holistic Health.* But when I visited the ashram, it was still in its early stages. About thirty-five people lived there, in a secluded valley in the lush Blue Mountains. They were surrounded by pine forests, lakes, meadows and streams. They grew most of their own vegetables in an organic garden on the grounds. All who lived there and all who visited enjoyed the same healthy vegetarian diet.

When I arrived at the ashram, I was greeted with the Sanskrit words, "J'ai bhagwan." This means, "I honor the divine within you." I came to learn that this beautiful greeting was always used at the ashram in lieu of hello and good-bye. This loving acknowledgement of one

---

*The Kripalu Center is now in the Berkshires. Its address is Box 793, Department ML, Lenox, Massachusetts 01240.

another sets the atmosphere for treating everyone in a kind, loving manner. It serves as a constant reminder of who each of us is and that there is a place in everyone that exemplifies the higher qualities of the human heart and spirit.

I arrived at the ashram just before satsang, which is a gathering of all the residents every evening to discuss anything that might come up. There were several residents who worked outside the ashram in Philadelphia. They brought up a variety of interesting situations for discussion. Plus there were always challenges and situations concerning ashram living that made for lively exchanges. Amrit commented often during these sessions, sharing his knowledge of teachings from the great masters as well as his own wisdom.

At my first satsang, Amrit spoke of the meaning of yoga. He said, "In its simplest meaning, yoga is finding happiness within ourselves by finding our inner core, our center and our inner/outer balance." He spoke of the power of love. "Nobody should ever hate anyone for any reason. You cannot hurt anyone else without hurting yourself first. No man in all of history has found contentment from only wealth, power or sensual pleasure." Uncovering our true sense of love and giving it freely is the basis for all we really want and need, he said. It is the basis for acceptance and love to be returned. Amrit also spoke of the life force, prana, that flows inside us. In the following days, I heard a lot more about prana — how to store it up, how to give it to others, how others can rob us of it.

Simply being in the presence of Amrit made me feel serene and uplifted. His manner was calm, modest, gentle, spiritual and loving. He seemed to be more of a holy man than anyone I had ever encountered. I had never seen anyone more at peace with himself.

My next morning at the ashram began with meditation, followed by instruction in yogic breathing, relaxation and asanas. I had never meditated. I did not know much about the practice, and I had never been very curious or interested. Meditation always had a religious connotation to me. If anyone had told me that I would some day make meditation a daily part of my life, I would have laughed at the notion. Sitting still, or just sitting quietly, was excruciating for me. When I tried to sit straight, I was very uncomfortable. I didn't realize how my posture had suffered because of MS. I did my best to keep my balance. I participated in the meditation sessions every day, trying to add a few minutes each day until I could sit straight and still for at least ten to fifteen minutes. The relaxation exercises that I learned at the ashram helped my meditation posture.

It was quite a revelation to me to see that I could actually control my bodily functions on demand. All I had to do was give a suggestion to a body part to quiet down and relax, and it complied. Amazing. Of course, we have all been able to hold our need to urinate until we could get to a bathroom. But at the ashram, I actually learned to control and quiet down the spasm in my leg, to discipline restless feelings and anxious stressful bodily reactions.

There has been much research on the effects of meditation and relaxation techniques since the days when I was first at the ashram. Ample scientific documentation exists on the positive effects of those techniques. Meditation and relaxation can be used instead of drugs to lower blood pressure and to eliminate pain and stress. We may be reluctant to believe how much our thoughts affect our body, but all we have to do is spend some time hooked to a biofeedback machine to begin understanding the power of suggestion.

The discovery that my thoughts had a profound effect on my body was one of the most impressive and important things I learned on my journey into health and healing. It was the key to convincing me to make a concerted effort to be conscious of all my thoughts and beliefs. The messages that the mind gives to the body will inevitably work changes at the cellular level.

When we began our breathing exercises on my first full day at the ashram, I wondered why we were bothering with such a self-evident practice. I had never paid much attention to my breathing. I figured that as long as I was alive, I must be breathing. What more could I want to learn about it? Breathing seemed to be a boring subject, something we all do automatically. Why think about it? It was just another one of those bodily functions that does not require any thought.

Wrong.

At the ashram, I learned that breathing is a way to bring the universe inside ourselves. It is really a fascinating function once you take a deeper look at it. As babies, we breathe properly. We know instinctively how to get what we need from breathing. Somewhere along the way, however, as we begin to grow up, our minds begin to overrule our good instincts. We let other pressures influence the way we breathe. Our minds habitually foul up the wonderful, body-smart way we breathed at birth. When the chest is constricted with daily emotions and stresses, it is difficult to breathe properly. We all need to stop and take a few deep, slow breaths to renew the connection between ourselves and the universe, to pull in the gift of energy that the universe is constantly offering. Deep, slow breathing is nature's tranquilizer and energizer. The breath is an indispensable aid in carrying on the work of health and homeostasis.

I was learning so much. I was beginning to revere the body that I had once taken so for granted. As we moved into the session on yogic postures, I gloried in all the discoveries I was making about myself. In the beginning, I could not do any of the postures during the hathayoga class at the ashram. As I watched the instructor, I became keenly aware of my limitations. I did what I could, however. And I listened and learned.

Looking around at the others practicing the postures, I thought, *I am the only one here at the ashram with an obvious handicap. Whoops. Cancel that negative. I mean I'm the only one with a physical challenge. What am I doing here anyway?*

Then the cheerleader who lives in my head kicked in: *Oh, honey, you have a right to be here. That's just your ego talking, just because you can't keep up. Everyone has a disability — I mean challenge — of some kind. It's just more obvious with some. So don't get hung up. Simply try to accept and learn from the great gift surrounding you.*

It felt so good to lighten up. The loving atmosphere at the ashram was so contagious that I could actually feel a shift within, a more tolerant, accepting attitude toward myself. I was beginning to appreciate myself more, to actually acknowledge all of my efforts, and perhaps even to accept myself as I am, just where I am. Feeling at peace, I took a deep breath and settled down to enjoy all the heavenly movement around me.

I stayed at the ashram for two weeks. During that time, I came to accept that my healing would be complete sooner or later. So much of what I heard there was what I had needed to hear for years. So much had opened up to me and in me and all around me. Everyone was so open, so honestly herself or himself, so serene, so accepting. I felt I had been given a privileged glimpse of our true nature, and it was magnificent. Yes, people can live and work with love and peace in their hearts and on their tongues. People can be in touch with their humanity first. They can be genuine, true, loving, peaceful and pure.

I felt like a child learning about the world for the first time. Yet, here I was a forty-nine-year-old homemaker, wife and mother of three. I used to spend my free time in community causes. Now I was spending time at what was commonly referred to, by the uninformed, as some "new age or occult" ashram. I was the oldest person at the ashram. I was physically handicapped. But I had refused to come to a halt because of a degenerative paralysis, a devastating prognosis and an uninformed medical community. I was opening up to new experiences, accepting change and reaching inside myself for answers that I could not find in my outer world.

Many of my fellow residents at the ashram were young adults whose parents no doubt had many mistaken impressions and who would have been thrilled to know of the invaluable lessons and sustaining values that their kids were experiencing. These kids arrived at the ashram bereft of meaning in their lives and out of touch with their own spirituality. For the first time, they could understand and relate to their own religious backgrounds, regardless of what they were; they found meaning and made wonderful sense out of everything at the ashram.

Amrit's wise offerings guided us all. "Your degree of fulfillment depends upon how deeply you are established in your own center, how consciously you are connected with your inner source of satisfaction," he told us. Being centered means that mind, heart, soul and body appropriately share in the work that we are doing. Living in our inner center means being grounded within ourselves; it means that our inner and outer selves are in harmony. What we really want from life, we must acknowledge, essentially comes from within us.

Amrit's words and messages went straight to my heart. His teachings were so reassuring to me, so in sync with what I needed to hear. It was like hearing what the knowing inside of me already knows. My strength will come from living what I learn as well as from what I already know.

Amrit often said, "When you do not accept yourself, nothing coming toward you is acceptable, not even love. When you are not feeling good about yourself, anything that is given to you — love, caring, understanding, acceptance — is not available to you. Your inner center, that which makes all experience of satisfaction possible, only comes into focus through self-acceptance. It goes out of focus through self-rejection."

So profound! How I needed to hear that. What are the subtle, insidious ways that I have suffered self-rejection? How have I ignored my inner self? How have I neglected my true, spiritual nature? I would always remember Amrit's words: "Your inner center, that which makes all experience of satisfaction possible, only comes into focus through self-acceptance. It goes out of focus through self-rejection."

Many times at the ashram I was overcome with the depth of it all. During one of those times, I had scribbled a poem on a napkin, trying to describe what I felt:

GURU AMRIT DESAI

At first I knew who you were
And who was I.
This evening was a blissful surprise
Through naked gaze, surrender and oneness,
The power of love reflected in eyes,
Love and energy coming through.

Some shake, some sigh, some shudder, some
    laugh.
I cry — in gratitude.
Your divine presence, a symbol of love,
The chanting, the flowers. The ecstasy of touching
    the love from within,
Feeling at one with the ABOVE.
I have written and I have erased. Words are out of
    place.
Words do not fit. A feeling is a feeling is a feeling.
THIS IS IT!
Writing these words forces me to think.
Sad to abandon my feelings. I blink and blink and
    blink.
What is reality?

As I left the ashram after my delicious two weeks, I
knew I would return to hear "J'ai bhagwan" again. I felt
more at one with myself than I ever had before. I felt a
renewed orientation to life. I had new-found liberation,
freedom and joy in permitting myself the luxury of not
worrying about anyone else. Just being me was so
exhilarating that it obliterated any of the anxiety I had
previously felt regarding my focused endeavor to regain
my health.

At one point during my stay, I had asked Amrit how
to incorporate all we experienced at the ashram into
our lives when we returned to the outside world. I
wondered how we could explain the transformations
that had occurred in us. He told me that there was no
need to try to convert anyone to anything or to try to
defend or explain too much. If asked about the ashram
— and only if asked — I should just try to explain in the
simplest way possible and only as much as is asked for,
since this is living our basic nature of simplicity and
love. He advised me just to continue in my spiritual

growth by treating everyone and everything with love and caring, especially myself. All love and caring expands from feeling it for ourselves first. If you love yourself, you will experience a serenity that is contagious. He said to endeavor always to do and say what we feel is good and right in our hearts. Then things will unfold the way they should. Being a good example is the best gift you can give anyone.

The First Shaky Steps
Toward Autonomy

*Most of us live by habit. We have not
always consciously made the choices that
shape our lives. We may even be unaware
of all of our options for choice. An illness
may sometimes represent an opportunity
to begin to live more consciously and
deliberately. By focusing people's attention
on their choices through the pain and
limitation they are causing, diseases may
give people both the chance to become
aware of these choices and the motivation
to act and make change where and when it
is needed. Through a process like this, we
may directly experience, for the first time,
the effect of our choices on our lives.*

> — Dr. Naomi Remen *in* The Human
> Patient

I couldn't wait to get home from the ashram.
I was so eager to share my realizations and experiences
with my husband, the only person who knew the depth
of my dilemma and all that I had been going through. I
wanted to tell him about the profound healing effect
the ashram had in my life. It took away any doubts I
had that I was doing the right things to improve my
health. I had so much to be thankful for, and I felt

grateful and forward-looking. My balance was better. I felt more energetic and had more strength in my hands and other areas of my body. I was still limping and dragging my right foot, but that seemed almost inconsequential.

I thought that my husband would feel good about what was happening for me, if only for the fact that this would ultimately affect him and our lives in a most positive way. I was so eager to share the distance I had just traveled, the depth of emotional, mental and spiritual experiences, the unmasking of my authentic inner self, the going home, the going within.

My husband met me at the airport. We embraced, and he suddenly made a move to be on our way. He seemed to be in a big hurry, so I limped along as quickly as I could to pick up my luggage and get going. It was good to see him. I smiled warmly as I tried to catch his eye. "It's good to see you," I said. "How are you?"

"Fine."

"How are the kids?"

"Fine."

"What's going on at home?"

"Nothing."

"Anything happening at work?"

"No."

Through all this, I tried to make some eye contact with him, but he wasn't having any of it. I was beginning to feel uneasy and stifled by his distancing manner and brusque responses. We got in the car without his ever once initiating a word of conversation or even asking how I was feeling or what was going on with me. Perhaps all the beautiful, high-spirited, emotion-packed memories I had of the ashram had blinded me, lulled me into a false sense of emotional security with my husband, lulled me into being so naive as to think I could share this important turning point in my life with him, that he would even be interested.

Watching him as we drove along, I couldn't help but break the silence by asking again, "Is anything the matter? What's wrong? Are you really okay?"

"Fine."

I thought, *If you are really fine, why don't you tell your face? It looks pretty dismal to me.* But I took the obvious hint, said nothing and rode along quietly. Once we got into the house, his very first words to me were, "Why are you limping, I mean, dragging your foot?"

WHAMMO!

I turned to face him and was hit with a full view of the disgust on his face. The blow was staggering. I felt the heat rising rapidly through my body. My hands felt clammy. My knees wobbled, and I sank into the nearest chair. Oh, how it hurt to have him look at me with eyes that saw and felt so little. *Why did he ask me that? What did he really mean by that question? What does he really want to know? I had been gone for only two weeks. He couldn't have forgotten how I walked when I left. He knew darn well why I was limping and dragging my foot. So why the question? Why the intimidating and belittling manner?*

I felt like I was losing that wonderful sense of self I had just acquired. It was slipping away so fast. I felt hurt and was real good at withdrawing and not sharing my pain. I can't remember ever allowing myself the luxury of expressing any hurt feelings directly (as though I couldn't permit myself to feel them). I was soon to learn how repressing and blocking my hurt and pain originated and why it developed into a full-blown habit. I wonder now how it would have felt to say spontaneously, "You're hurting my feelings." But those words did not occur to me at the time. Not only did I think that any adult should have realized how hurt I was; but I was hurting too much to react verbally. My long-time, self-defeating habit was to hold my feelings in, make some excuse for the other person and get over the hurt by myself.

Am I overreacting to his question? Why am I being overly sensitive to something to which I should be accustomed? He often comes up with some unfortunate choice of words, but usually covers it up with some clever or witty disguise that makes me laugh. I was well aware that he dealt with anger, frustration or anxiety in this manner. And I had become very creative in intellectualizing my hurt feelings away. But somehow nothing felt the same to me on the day I got home from the ashram. I couldn't dismiss that intimidating voice, the look on his face, the insensitivity, the whole unanswerable, inane question. I was puzzled by my reaction. Why did his attitude continue to take me by surprise? And why was I unable to disregard it this time?

My thoughts flashed back to an evening about two years before when we were on our way home from a friend's house. He was particularly uncommunicative the whole evening. After asking him several times if anything was wrong and getting no response, he finally told me: "Your illness turns me off."

I could not believe my ears. I immediately thought of all the effort I had put in, of all the years of constant support for his endeavors, of nursing him through his many illnesses and traumas. I thought of how little support I had ever gotten from him. Now, the very first time he was challenged to be there for me, he couldn't do it. He didn't even want to. How the heck could he even admit that to me?

I was too shocked to respond verbally at the time. Later I thought there was no point in responding. It still hurt to think that I meant so little to him. I felt a humiliation that was deeply imprinted on my soul. I began to view my world differently, to see myself through his eyes. And now this exchange. His whole demeanor from the time he met me at the airport had been aimed at putting distance between us. His question served to put the finishing touches on shutting me out. He knew (perhaps unconsciously) that his question was demeaning, that he was displaying his power by being intimidating and showing up my imperfection. What a classic example of interaction between spouses. Worst of all, this is how far too many couples think they are resolving their conflicts — by denial and suppression, which only serve to compound the issues until they are too disguised and blown out of proportion to begin to deal with. The subtle and not-so-subtle ways in which we communicate are most revealing and deserve our consideration and understanding in all our relationships.

My husband's effect on me was amazing. Despite the recent satisfaction and comfort I had experienced from that beautiful glimpse into my higher self, I was buckling under, slipping away from my newly discovered center. At that point I was far from feeling any self-acceptance. I was, however, at least aware of what was happening, instead of totally denying and repressing my feelings. I was very well aware that I was permitting his attitude to create my reality. Like a giant blotter, I was soaking up his attitude and opinion. I was not only hurt by his remark, but I was also compounding my own suffering by my own self-rejection. I was relinquishing all my higher power to understand who I really am.

I knew that this was an important realization for me. My understanding of how we lose our inner connection by accepting what comes in at us, to the detriment of our spiritual nature, was new to me. How remarkable that this exchange with my husband was not so subtle and insidious, that it was obvious. I should have dealt with it directly in some constructive manner once I realized what it was. And yet, I didn't. I swallowed it. But not for long. There was a difference this time.

I tried to view his question from his perspective. *What was he really trying to express? What did he actually expect? Was I such a disappointment to him? Was he ashamed of me? Did I embarrass him?* I asked myself whether I was overreacting, reacting too negatively, feeling hurt for no reason, reading too much into this whole scene.

My sense of the ridiculous surfaced to rescue me. I managed a half-baked smile. *Incredible. I have not yet been away for a full day from the ashram — where I was surrounded by caring and love, well on my way to freedom, peace, higher consciousness, wisdom, enlightenment, nirvana — and I lose it all so quickly. I lose it because of my own attitude, one that I should have expected, confronted and refused to tolerate years ago.* I nearly laughed out loud at the thought of having worried over how to deal with others when obviously I was desperately in need of dealing with myself most of all.

Smiling inwardly to release some of the tension that was building, I was able to ask my husband in a somewhat normal tone, "Honey, can you help me to understand what you meant by the question you just asked me — you know, why was I limping and dragging my foot?"

He could hardly look at me as he mumbled, "Oh, I don't know. I was just noticing how you were walking and uh, uh, uh, uh . . . ." His voice trailed off. I knew there was no need to pursue this and that he was not feeling too good about it either. I also knew that something very important had just happened with me. As usual, the clarity and significance did not reveal itself until later. I was still trying to reason away all my hurts when I hugged my husband and told him I wanted to go upstairs to take a nap. As I laid in my bed, I went through all the possible excuses for his behavior. *After all, he was just being honest that time when he said my illness turned him off. So what? Don't most men feel that way? They don't know how to deal with illness and are not natural nurturers like women.* In my generation, men were not taught about nurturing and were not concerned with any caring or communication skills. Not until many years later did society help them become aware of how these gaps in their education affected their relationships.

Perhaps he hadn't meant to hurt me. Instead, he might have been expressing his own anxiety. Could he be hurting, too? Could he be feeling, "Why did she have to happen to me?" Could he be wondering how bad I would get? Maybe he felt helpless. Or maybe he just didn't know how to react to my illness. He probably didn't even know how to ask for help.

I felt sad for him when I realized that there could have been many reasons behind his remark. *He could have been expecting a total cure. He could have forgotten how bad my limp was when I left for the ashram. He could have been a victim of denial who was just seeing the disability for the first time.*

I decided that I would see him as being a little perplexed and not knowing quite how to deal with his confusion. Whatever the motivation behind his remark, it simply did not matter any more. I was relieved to be telling myself that my illness could not have been easy for him either and that his words might not have been meant to hurt me at all.

I was ready to sleep when a wee voice inside me said, *Stay with this, Rach. Pay attention. It is important to give this more thought, some kind of processing.*

So I looked at the situation from a different angle. I wondered if I still wanted to be perfect for my husband.

Did I feel less than whole? Did I feel guilty for getting sick? Was it my fault? Was it threatening to have him think I was disabled and that I could no longer take care of his many needs? Would this diminish my value in his eyes? Would he abandon me? Was I scared that I could no longer be Mrs. Fix-it for him because I was so desperately trying to fix myself? Am I the one who is feeling worthless, or is he telling me that I am no longer of any value?

Geez. Where does his thinking begin or end and where does mine begin and end? How did our thinking become so enmeshed that I can't distinguish which is whose?

It seemed I had become a mere reflection of everything my husband thought, of everything he felt and of everything he did. It was scary to realize how many of my husband's feelings I had taken on during our twenty-six years of marriage. I had abandoned my own feelings for the sake of a peaceful co-existence. I was the one who felt responsible for making the marriage work, and I refused to permit our differences to interfere. I simply had to make it all work. After all, isn't life just one adjustment after another? Nobody ever told me that the only permanently adjusted people are in the grave.

On the outside, I had seemed to be a separate person. I had my own interests all during my marriage. We didn't share many interests, in fact. But that was just my worldly self that was distinct from my husband. My inner self was being abused. I had ignored how much I was hurting inside. This, as much as anything else, was causing disease in my body. And now, the disease in my body was jolting me into the realization that I needed to reclaim myself.

I wonder how many women of my generation can identify with my long-standing assumption that my spouse's opinion of me was the truth about who I was. If his opinion was negative, then I was nothing. I never thought to view his attitude toward me as a reflection of his own uneasiness about himself and of his inability to confront his own issues.

Younger women, those of my daughter's generation, seem to be very creative about satisfying and nurturing themselves. They seem more real, more themselves, more honestly assertive and healthier. In their relationships, they do not hold back their feelings until everything blows up. They do not deny their feelings. They seem to understand that they are autonomous individuals who may choose to come together in a relationship. Their ultimate goal is to be one when they are together while helping each other grow and become whole when they are apart. They know that it is impossible to be a successful WE until each partner is a successful ME. The healthiest relationships are with two autonomous selves. Fortunately, it's never too late to learn this lesson.

I had just come from the mountain top, from a higher place that brought me back to my true self (a place I had experienced often in my youth but which had become hidden under life's pressures on the way to adulthood). At the ashram, I had unmasked my higher self. My problem before was that I had not been looking high enough.

The years of my marriage had undermined my self-confidence. I had invested myself heavily in someone whose attitudes and values were completely out of sync with my own. I realized that I had absolutely no need to prove myself to my husband or to wish his attitude different. The simple truth was that we were two very different people. I was getting to the point where I could honestly accept him for who he was without buying into his feelings or permitting those feelings to violate me in any way.

It was understanding how crucial the acknowledgement of my needs and feelings was that made me dare to risk becoming an autonomous self. As I lay on my bed, I had the sensation that I was experiencing a separation from my husband. I was leaving the US and the WE and coming into my own. I was becoming an autonomous ME.

Even this giant step forward in my thinking, however, did not seem to carry me far enough. That small voice that had urged me to process all my feelings after my husband's hurtful remark was not satisfied. It urged me to continue processing.

I went back to my insatiable need to fulfill my husband's needs. Where did that come from? *What was I afraid of that made the role of indispensable caretaker seem the only one possible for me? Would my husband leave me if I could not perform as before? It was not in my nature to fear being abandoned. Or was it?* I was surprised to even consider being abandoned at this point. The fear had surfaced, though, and I had to question seriously what my real insecurities were and why I was feeling them so strongly now.

There seemed to be something deep inside of me that was surfacing slowly. It was screaming to come out. I felt like I was being tested and challenged to the limit and depth of my very essence. I felt like a tea bag that had to be thrown into hot water to realize its own strength.

I knew that repressing my needs and feelings for so long had caused the kind of cumulative stress that made me vulnerable to disease. Now the disease seemed almost like a gift. It woke me up, and there was no going back. I could no longer endure any wounds behind a smile. We forfeit our very being when we deny or ignore our feelings. Those feelings feed us much-needed information that can have a profound impact on our lives.

I knew I had to confront my own deeper reasons for denying and avoiding my needs and feelings. *Why hadn't I dealt with my situation sooner? Why during twenty-six years of marriage had I refused to challenge my husband for his obvious put-downs of me? Why did it have to take MS to get my attention, to let me know what I was doing to myself?* My illness was forcing me to face my life and just how out of balance it was, how I was living someone else's life, according to his needs and desires. Somehow, I needed MS in my life to show me the importance of my own needs, issues and inner self.

I began to wonder why I was attracted to extremely needy people in the first place. I always seemed to be living vicariously by fixing life for others. I was Mrs. Fix-it for everyone. Even as a young child, I was the caretaker in my family. When the others spoke up for what they needed or wanted, it always surprised me they could be so bold. I could never do that. I do not think I was unhappy about this. I always had the feeling that I should be satisfied with whatever I got or with whatever happened and go about the business of helping and pleasing others. I simply went along thinking that this was the right thing to do. I don't recall feeling that I had any problems or really needed anything. I was so focused on taking care of others that any other feeling I might have was soon diminished. I got my identity from outside myself. I got my value and satisfaction from people-pleasing.

But why was I like that as a child? And why did I remain stuck in that role as an adult? I knew that I had to get to the core of my existence to bring out the unconscious reasons for my drive to be so needed. I knew that any changes in my life had to begin with me. *I am the only one over whom I have any control. I have the power to create my own reality. Why have I created this one of the need to be needed?*

I felt as if I were on to something big. I knew that I was dealing with some universal issues. I had come down with a serious, life-threatening illness so that I would place my attention where it belonged — on my own life and needs rather than on fixing life for others. It was not the disease of multiple sclerosis that I so urgently needed to overcome; it was the extreme need to be needed. *What did I believe and accept from the earliest messages I had gotten in my life that set me up to assume that my value depended upon how successful I was at taking care of others. How was I set up to lose all boundaries and to develop great tolerance for injustices to myself, as long as I felt indispensable?*

Again I felt the contrast of being at the ashram, where for the very first time I could let go of any external focus and open up to what I really felt rather than what I told myself I should feel. The old tyranny of the shoulds had begun to slip away at the ashram. I had felt the freedom to feel and speak my heart, without censorship, without fear of hurt or risk of rejection. I had never felt more real and at one with my inner self, more whole and more alive. I had never experienced such an atmosphere of unconditional love and acceptance. As soon as I was greeted with "J'ai bhagwan," I knew that all feeling and communication would be coming from and directed to the higher self in each one of us there. Gone was the need to explain, to defend or to seek approval. All of us just knew that unconditional love and acceptance were ours automatically because we were there at the ashram.

What a feeling that was. I was reminded of what the *Course in Miracles* implies — that there are two kinds of people. There are those who are coming from a place of love and those who are coming from a place of needing love. The only way to respond to either type is in a loving, caring way. The one question to ask yourself, when you are uncertain about how to respond, is: "What is the loving thing to do? Or what is the loving thing to say?"

But I was digressing. I was resisting a confrontation with the real issue of why I had to stifle my own feelings and needs in deference to others, why my worth was always at the mercy of others. *If I wasn't needed, I might be abandoned. Why did I always have to be there for others, no matter how tired or stressed I felt?* Until I knew that I had MS, I was always too busy, busy, busy with others to notice how run down and stressed out I was. I laughed with self-recognition as I recalled some lines from e.e. cummings: "If you can be, be ... If not, cheer up and go on about other people's business, doing and undoing unto others, 'til you drop."

But my predicament wasn't funny. My mood turned sad again as I wondered how I had let myself down. *Why had I added insult to injury by belittling myself for having a disability? Geez. For a time there, I didn't even have me to fall back on for support.* Amrit's words came back to me: "Your inner center, that which makes all experience of satisfaction possible, only comes into focus through self-acceptance. It goes out of focus through self-rejection."

I was beginning to feel awful. I just could not tolerate the thought that I would feel less worthy because I had multiple sclerosis. I could not accept that I had so little sense of myself that I took on some of my husband's attitude, which made me feel flawed somehow. This was too much. I couldn't stand it.

I got out of bed to pour some cool water on my face. As I looked up from the basin, I caught my reflection in the bathroom mirror. I heard myself say out loud, "I really do love you, you know." We smiled at each other, my reflection and I. It felt good. I thought I should say things like that to myself more often. *That's not a bad idea, Rach. I need to do something to keep the thought of loving my body in my consciousness. That's the least I can do since I've spent so many years giving myself negative messages. In fact, that is exactly what I will do. Every night, before I go to bed, I'll look in the mirror and tell myself that I love my body unconditionally.*

With that resolution made, I climbed back into bed and decided to let myself sleep. I knew I had not probed deeply enough into my need to be needed. But at least I had defined the problem. I knew I was on the right track. Rest would probably help me more than anything else at the moment. I had to remember the needs of my body, a body that was improving and working for me in many ways, one that was responding and recuperating.

The Joy of Real Connection

For the next five nights, I kept my resolution to tell my body that I loved it unconditionally. The first night, when I looked in the mirror and said, "I love you unconditionally," I did not really feel involved. The next night, when I looked in the mirror and tried to make meaningful eye contact, I felt a little ridiculous. But a promise is a promise. "I love you unconditionally," I said out loud. I kept at it, and on the fifth night, when I looked in the mirror, I saw real eyes looking back at me for the first time. I said, "I love you unconditionally," and I really felt the words as I moved in closer to that wonderful pair of eyes looking back at me. I said, "You know, I really do love every inch of you." I felt my nose pressing against the mirror. I guess I just couldn't get close enough. I blew myself a kiss and went to bed.

That night, sleep would not come. I was feeling the heavy sadness again. Before long, the dam burst wide open. I was crying uncontrollably for that hurting inner self that I had lost touch with, that I had abandoned. I had forsaken my whole being and become just a human doing instead of a human being. I didn't even recognize when I was stressed out.

People who love themselves, who have a balance between their inner and outer selves, are very clear on what they feel and what they need. Their basis of focus, their whole sense of who they are, is inside themselves. It is not about whether somebody else approves; it is about doing one's best, within one's own honesty and integrity, within one's own values. The healthy person feels validated as a human being, not as an achiever, a goal setter or a producer.

The old questions persisted: *Where and how did I get so off track? How had I gotten so out of touch with me?* I came from a very kind and loving family. I could remember no major tragedy that might have been traumatizing. *Why did I need to make myself so indispensable to others?*

Why didn't I get the message earlier? Why didn't I confront the fact that my husband had so many problems of his own that he was incapable of dealing with me or any of my needs? Did I contribute to this by going along with it, by being undemanding and passive? All I wanted to do was keep the peace and not be a burden. Why didn't I deal with the fact that he was emotionally unavailable most of the time? Why had I settled for merely hiding my hurt feelings behind some socially acceptable cover of pleasantness, behind a smile, a joke, laughter. This had been my custom since childhood.

Why? Why? Why?

Once again, I got up and looked in the mirror. I noticed my expression softening as I felt the love welling up inside me, sweet love for that hurting, child-like reflection looking back at me. As I continued to gaze at myself, longing to make a deeper connection, the sweetest, clearest, purest eyes were looking back at me, touching me deeply with their child-like innocence. They were the most beautiful and loving eyes imaginable. I felt a shiver weaving up my spine as a haunting hint of sadness and longing held me spellbound.

Gently brushing aside a tear, I said lovingly, "I know you weren't really left on the doorstep in a basket. You really were loved, and no one could ever have abandoned you that way. That was just a silly joke. Of course. Surely. It was just a silly joke."

I felt nearly overwhelmed with tenderness and wonder. "Oh, my goodness," I said, "you really are in there. Aren't you? You're always there for me in that deep place that never changes. Aren't you? You wonderful one. How sweet it is to be loved by you."

Oh, God, what a feeling! What joy to feel some real connection again. How did I ever let myself get so separated from this necessary, wholesome connection, which makes everything else not just tolerable, but welcome?

Going Home to the Ashram

Unless you come from a place where you have had some real exceptional luck in your upbringing, you come out of a family that has rules that shame feelings, needs and wants. So many families won't let children express their feelings. Feelings are there in order to give the brain a way to adjust to new reality . . . expressing anger, sadness, joy, fear. Our emotions are part of our personal power. Our fear is part of our wisdom. This is the way we complete things so we can be present. We complete the past so that we can be present. Sadness is like grief. Sadness is a healing feeling. Anger is our protector. When you deny people feelings, you deny them power.

— John Bradshaw in his television series,
Bradshaw on the Family

I felt consumed by the need to do some deep reflective work. Things seemed to be coming together in my mind, to be fitting better. But there was a big chunk missing, something crucial that would not surface. Maybe my defenses against pain were trying to protect me, as usual. But I had come too far; there was no going back.

I felt blocked. I felt trapped. It occurred to me that home might not be the best place to do the kind of soul-searching that I needed to do. There was enough resistance on my part without all the distractions at home. When I was at home, I slipped too easily back into old habits. I didn't want to chance losing myself again in the status quo.

Naturally, I thought of the ashram. That loving, supportive environment would help me make the changes I wanted in my health and in my life. Silence and aloneness were always available there. Introspection and self-love were a way of life.

Because of long-standing repression, I knew that I had some heavy-duty pain and sadness to pull up and work through. There was simply no other way for me. I had to be alone. I had to dig out the root causes, to feel the hurt and the pain of my inner child. I had to be able to feel as bad as I really feel, in order to acknowledge, grieve over and let go of whatever it was that was having such a basic effect on my personality.

When I arrived back at the ashram and heard the "J'ai bhagwan" greeting once again, I felt at home, at peace and at one with myself immediately. I was very much at ease and ready to let whatever come through, to let go and let the flow happen.

Early one morning, just after I had taken a long walk around the grounds, I had the opportunity to get to the kind of work I needed to do. The air was crisp, and the sun was beginning to dry the dew on the grass. I sat down on that beautiful green carpet that seemed to go on forever. There was no one around. I sat there, feeling the gift of life, letting the warm sun envelop me completely.

My interior monologue began: *What do I really need? I think it is great to be a nurturing caretaker, to understand compromise and flexibility, if such a role is a choice and not a duty.* I was too aware now that my fix-it mentality and my need to feel responsible for others were rooted in my childhood. Such behavior was the primary way I had gotten approval as a child. Becoming a people-pleaser didn't seem very much like a choice to me. It was more like a duty, even a compulsion.

It didn't take long before those sweet, innocent eyes I had seen in the mirror were with me again. I felt the same overwhelming sadness. I don't know for how long, but I just sat there surrendering to the sadness and crying my heart out. In a quietly tearful voice, I said, "I need guidance. I know there is a higher power operating in this universe and operating in me. Please, please, please, make your presence known to me. Help me through this maze."

I heaved a deep sigh and wept more and more. I felt the letting go, the giving in, the helpless surrender, as I crumbled into a lump on the ground. All the tension drained from my body. I let it all go as I wept.

After a long time, I slowly began to uncurl my body, stretching it out on the grass. I felt weak and limp, but at the same time I was flooded with a warm, healing energy. I got up and walked over to a tree. I put my arms around that tree and stood there hugging it. I felt its aliveness. I had a strong sense of really caring about that tree. It was so good to be alone with my arms around that tree. I felt myself melting into it so that the tree and I were one. I felt stronger and more caring about myself, too. I whispered confidently: "You are going to be all right." I meant that no matter what happened, it would be right for me.

Before long, those sad eyes surfaced again. This time I recalled something I had said to those eyes in the mirror at home. The words came back to me: *I know you weren't really left on the doorstep in a basket. You really were loved and no one could ever have abandoned you that way. That was just a silly joke. Of course. Surely. It was just a silly joke.* Odd that I should remember those words as I stood clinging to a tree. I thought about my siblings and my parents and how lucky I was to have been brought up in such a nice family. I thought of my mother, with whom I was particularly close. I thought of all the meaningful talks I had with her; they had continued even after her death. I looked up to the top of the tree and felt like a tiny child beside it. When my thoughts rolled back to my family, that deep, tormenting sadness welled up inside me again. It was so puzzling. I could not understand why I was feeling sad when I was remembering how well I had always been treated. In fact, I had never had a spanking, never even been yelled at. Well, I guessed that wasn't surprising. *Why should anyone be angry with me when I was always trying so hard to please them? I never did anything to risk anyone's getting angry with me. My entire life was geared toward finding ways to please and help.*

I wondered why my need to be wanted and needed was so different from my sister's or my brother's. *What was it about me that made me such a caretaker? Why weren't they the same way?*

Then it all came crashing into place: *But I'm not an orphan. I know darn well I'm not an orphan.* I tightened my arms around that tree and held on for dear life, crying. *I know for sure that I definitely was not adopted. They were just kidding. Did I actually believe them? Of course not. How could I? No, I couldn't have believed that I was found on the doorstep in a basket. Or did I? I know very well why they told me that. I know exactly why they said that. They certainly explained it enough times as I got older. And we all laughed and joked about it.*

As very young children automatically and sponta-neously go into and out of the alpha state, somewhere between fantasy and reality, I must have hooked into and believed what my sister and brother were telling people. It all began when I was just a tot, when it was hard to know where truth began and storytelling left off. I could just see myself as I was then — a toddler with pale golden hair, walking between my older brother and sister, each of them holding one of my hands as we made our way down the street. Because I was a towhead and did not look a bit like either one of them, my brother and sister were often asked, "Who is that little shiksa you're always taking care of?" They soon tired of the question and concocted a story of their own to give as a stock answer. "Oh, her. We found her on the doorstep in a basket." They would laugh. Their joke about how I was found in a basket continued for years. But I knew it was a joke. I knew it was not true. OR DID I?

It seems that I must have believed it to some degree, on some level. Surely, it is conceivable that I would believe it in that state of childhood where the imagination runs free, where fact and fantasy are one. But when we laughed about it during family stories when I was a teenager, it never occurred to me that somewhere deep in my subconscious, the story took hold. I accepted and believed it. My subconscious belief that I was an orphan affected my sense of self-worth and, therefore, my attitudes and behaviors throughout my life. It was both alarming and incomprehensible to me that I could possibly still be carrying the scars of this well-intentioned story, the scars of having been abandoned by my real parents, of not being loved or wanted, of not belonging. A wave of shame came over me, and I had to admit that I grew up with the vague feeling of being ashamed most of the time. But I never understood why. It would make sense that if I thought I was found in a basket on the doorstep, I would feel that I had done something shameful to merit having been abandoned by my biological parents. It must have been my fault that they could not love me or want me.

Shame makes us feel inadequate or phony and bad. The underlying feeling that others may see through our facade, that they may find out how ashamed we feel and then how flawed and defective we are, is usually behind the need to people-please. No wonder I could not afford to show any anger or negative feelings. After all, I should be eternally grateful that I had been taken in, cared for and fed. I was bad enough to have been abandoned. I learned early to repress and to deny my real feelings since I had no rights. Feelings are a barometer of what's happening to us. I was numbing myself in order not to feel them.

As I held on to that cool, soothing tree, I could remember some very early feelings of shame and humiliation at having to accept food and lodging — handouts — because I didn't rightfully belong. Therefore, I had to do something to deserve all the kindness I was getting. Using my survival instincts, I knew that being available and a good caretaker would make me needed, even indispensable and would serve to give me value. It would also serve to help me feel that I was contributing something, that I was not quite so beholden.

Life, when understood, is always a neat package. What I had accepted and believed from my early programming set me up to be attracted to and to attract people who were very needy in some way. If I could fix it for others, I would have value. I would feel worthy. Developing caretaking skills became my goal as a youngster. I desperately needed to work at belonging and feeling worthy. I worked hard and became an expert at it. The fix-it personality was a role I learned early and grew into comfortably. Nevertheless, it was still a role. It did not come from the real me. It came from what I believed about myself. It gave me an external focus. I never lived my own life. I was out of touch with what I was really feeling because I was so busy doing and being for others. Everyone else had to come first. I believed I was doing the right thing. But, in fact, by being excessively nurturing, guess who I got to avoid? ME.

Of course, I thought I was doing the right thing by happily being of service and taking care of whatever was needed by others. As I got older, I became more and more oblivious to what a healthy person's number one priority has to be — her own needs. Eventually, all the real feelings that I had stuffed away where I wouldn't have to face them found a way to get my attention. They made me sick, literally. I had never realized that the stress that comes from denying our own needs and feelings is incredible and cumulative. In my opinion, this stress is at the root of most addictions and illnesses. I had been numbing out my needs and feelings for years. When I got sick, what was my first symptom? Numbness. An interesting correlation between how a disease manifested itself in my physical body and what I had been doing to my psyche. When I was told that I had multiple sclerosis and when I realized that I was deteriorating to the point where I could not do much for myself, let alone others, I could no longer ignore myself and all those needs I had been denying for years.

I am now aware of what an enormous amount of energy it takes to live in denial of real feelings, energy that is robbed from other body systems. I also know that the emotion we suppress does not go away. Translated, emotion is E-motion, meaning, E=energy in motion. If the emotion or feeling is important and we ignore it often or we cannot find a way to express it constructively, the energy gets trapped and causes a blockage somewhere in the body. This trapped energy can be the cause of any number of maladies.

When I was living in constant need of pleasing others, I became very adept at picking up all the non-verbal clues about how others were feeling and what they were needing. Being married to a needy man helped me perpetuate the pattern and allowed me to stay in my comfort zone. But I never received the appreciation and value I expected. Not being appreciated only made me escalate my efforts, work all the harder to fulfill his needs. I ignored my own needs to such an extent that I got multiple sclerosis. Then my own needs became so crucial to my survival that I had to give them priority. MS was the heaven-sent vehicle, the gift that told me I was stressing myself to death. I had to do all and be all. I couldn't say no. I couldn't ask for help. MS made sure that I could no longer do unto others.

I was beginning truly to appreciate the whole process. I will be forever grateful that I was intuitively led to view my diagnosis of MS as both a crisis and an opportunity. It was an opportunity to go within and to understand the depth of what I was all about. It was an opportunity to learn some of the secrets of the universe and my relationship to it, to know and appreciate the authentic me.

I realized I was still clinging to the tree planted in the broad green lawn at the ashram. I marveled at the remarkable range of emotions that I had experienced in such a short time. I had no idea what would happen or how it would come out. I only knew that these buried emotions had to surface and be dealt with or they would manifest elsewhere in my body again and again until I learned the lesson that I could care for no other person successfully until I took care of my own needs first.

I have since been told that what I put myself through that morning at the ashram is known as grief work. The grief was for my hurting inner child, whose pain had never been acknowledged and never worked through. This, no doubt, is why I felt that I had to permit myself the opportunity not to cover up any longer, to let myself feel as bad as I felt, to get into the depth of feeling as low as possible, to let it all out. Grief is an honest emotion. We need to recognize and feel it in order to get past it, let it go and continue with our lives. I realized that by avoiding the sadness and not going through the grief work, by pushing it away as I had done for years, I was actually pushing myself away from me. I thought I could rise above all that. Nonsense!

Everyone has experienced grief, not just through the death of someone dear but also through change. We grieve over change. To have a beginning, we have to experience an ending. To the degree that we can permit ourselves to grieve, we can accept change and growth.

I was grieving for more than just my hurt, neglected inner child. I was grieving over the end of a co-dependent relationship as well. I was grieving at having made another step toward the change I wanted, toward the state of being an autonomous self.

I stepped back from the tree and wrapped my arms around myself. I felt like I was hugging that small child within. It felt so good! When we heal our memories, it is no trivial matter. We are not playing games; we are not making believe. The healing is real.

I GOT IT. FINALLY, I GOT IT!

Letting Go of the Shame by Sharing It

My time of self-discovery under the tree at the ashram was only part of my journey toward wholeness. I had discovered my shame and its source and admitted it to myself. But I knew that I had to share the process. The evening satsang would be a fine place for such a sharing. I recalled how much I had appreciated hearing the others share their experiences.

As I walked back toward the ashram, I heard beautiful music. I flung my arms wide open and began to sway to the chords. My lack of coordination and poor balance brought me to an abrupt halt several times. But I swayed on. Nothing could rain on my parade or interrupt my spirit at that moment. I made myself a silent promise to be able to enjoy dancing with the same lovely balance and graceful movement that I once had so naturally, prior to the onset of MS.

I knew that I had to talk about my feelings, that working them through on my own would not be enough. The most effective way to get rid of deep shame (even shame that is unjustifiable and has no realistic basis, as is true of all shame that originates in early childhood) is to feel it, dig out the causes and understand how and why we took it on, then talk about it. Before we can let our shame go forever, we have to diminish the importance and significance we unwittingly attached to it. The most crucial aspect of shame is the absolute need to hide it and the reasons behind it. Shame is about isolation and hiding. So, of course, we must talk about it; we must share our shame with others in order to disperse it.

I had felt shame because I had erroneously concluded that I must have been so bad my real parents didn't want me. I believed they had abandoned me. I had tried to hide and overcome this shame by being a good little caretaker, working hard to gain the acceptance of the people who had taken me in. This unresolved childhood trauma had marked me for life. Finally I had uncovered it and exposed it for what it was. Surely, by sharing that process with others, I would be rid of the shame. Perhaps what I had to say would trigger messages from which everyone at the satsang could benefit.

Although I knew I had to share my discovery with others, I was apprehensive. I was so very unaccustomed to expressing my feelings or sharing my pain. Yet, I also knew that this was all the more reason for me to do so. What better place than the ashram to begin to integrate and put into practice all that I was learning.

That evening as I sat at the satsang among the others, I allowed myself to respond fully and completely to the feeling coming from all the care and love surrounding me. I felt honored and lucky to have found this place. I felt humble. At the first opening in the discussion, I heard myself saying that I had something difficult to share. Then the words just came rolling out. I was surprised at how smoothly and honestly I could name my shame. The people at the satsang responded to me. They asked questions and made interesting comments. They seemed to identify with my experience. The relief I felt was liberating. I felt good, very comfortable and peaceful. Is there a quicker road to glorious intimacy than a sharing of real feelings?

I was beginning to realize that feelings are the most helpful and necessary tools we have. Feelings give us vital information about how we relate to ourselves, to others and to the world in which we live. We understand how we perceive ourselves though our feelings. We know if our experiences are good or bad through our feelings. Feelings tell us when something needs our attention. Feelings are authentic and reliable. Denied and repressed feelings can get stuck in our bodies and cause energy blocks, circulatory problems and chronic stress.

Children are often told that they really do not feel what they are feeling. This causes them to repress their feelings, to distrust their real feelings. This leaves children even more vulnerable and dependent because the one reliable indicator they have — their feelings — has not been validated. Imagine their confusion and distrust. This can be the beginning of the lack of self-confidence and self-esteem that plagues people for the rest of their lives.

Parents do not intentionally deny a child's feelings. A child cries out, "It's dark in my bedroom and I'm scared." The anxious parent responds, "There's nothing to be scared of." Still, the child's real feeling of fright is dismissed. Better for the parent to say, "Yes, I understand that you're scared." Or, if the child says, "I want Oreo cookies," the parent, instead of saying, "No, you don't really want Oreo cookies" and denying the child's real desire for Oreos, should say, "Yes, I understand that you want Oreo cookies, but you can't have them right now." With the latter statement, the parent acknowledges the child's real feeling in a non-judgmental way but also tells the child that she cannot have whatever she wants. In this way, the child does not get the message that her feelings are bad or wrong, and she is not confused about her real feelings.

There are many subtle ways that we humans close ourselves off from each other. We do not make the effort to remain open to love from others because we are engaged subconsciously in an inner struggle to love and accept ourselves. If we cannot love ourselves, no matter how hard we look for acceptance outside ourselves, we will not find it. Love has to begin with love of the self. It cannot come from any other source.

Self-esteem happens naturally when we come to terms with who we authentically are. It cannot be verified by others. Only we can validate ourselves. When we understand our own worth, we communicate it eloquently to others, without speaking a word. Our good vibrations and peaceful demeanors automatically influence others to feel the same way about us as we do about ourselves. How we value ourselves is reflected in everything we do and say. The more positive we are about ourselves, the more positive we will be about others. The ability to respect and admire ourselves is a prerequisite for any relationship. Only to the extent that we care about and love ourselves can we care about and love others.

All my life, because of that one repeated message from early childhood, I had been giving away little pieces of myself, bit by bit. Finally, I had given away so much of myself that I had lost my own reality. When I began recovering my sense of self, I realized that we rarely do anything that is inconsistent with the mental picture we have of ourselves. Self-image is based on what we believe and accept as truth about ourselves; it is the very basis of personality. Every aspect of our behavior is affected by this self-image — our ability to relate to others, our choices, our capacity to grow and change, our skills, our perceptions, our attitudes. Authorities in the field of human behavior claim that a strong, positive self-image is the best possible assurance of a successful and happy life. Self-image controls everything we say or do. This makes it vitally important and well worth whatever effort is necessary to distinguish between old, hand-me-down beliefs and our own original, true and real thoughts about ourselves. The primacy of self-image also makes self-affirmation a necessity. I began affirming myself by accepting myself as a unique individual. *There is no other person in the world exactly like me. There is no need for comparison because I am uniquely me. I accept and love myself with all my imperfections. I know that I do not have to be perfect because I am perfectly me. I accept others with all of their imperfections. I release all negativity. I often think of all my good qualities, even those I have been hiding from myself. As I allow myself to become more aware of possessing these fine qualities, I will naturally display them to the benefit of myself, my loved ones and the whole world. The more I recognize the good qualities in myself, the more I will see them in others.*

The mind cannot focus on the negative and the positive at the same time. When I focus on the positive qualities in myself and others, I am not thinking negatively. I am free of fear, worry, hate and other negative thoughts. I am building a happier reality. By projecting love to others, I can appreciate the power of the boomerang effect. Smiles and sincere compliments are potent for me as I grow toward my true self-actualization.

After the beautiful, loving satsang at the ashram, I was relieved and exhilarated all at the same time, for having gone through so much and having let go of so much. I felt happy and satisfied that I had been able to accomplish that for which I had traveled again to the ashram. I experienced a great deal of aloneness at the ashram; that was one of the reasons I went there — to be alone without being lonely. For the first time in my life, I had found an absolutely safe environment in which I could feel and be my real self, no matter what that self felt like. I felt instant acceptance and unconditional love just for being a human, not for what I did or did not do. It was a place where I could be more honest about myself, without social censoring, than I ever thought possible. To be is all there is at the ashram.

The healing power of unconditional love is undeniable. It gives us the courage to be who we were born to be, rather than what our families and significant others expect us to be. My experience at the ashram helped me realize that I had not only the right but the obligation to be myself above all.

The injunction to "know thyself" is nearly as old as the human race. Socrates taught that self-knowledge is the basis of all knowledge. The wise Rabbi Zusya said shortly before his death, "In the world to come, I shall not be asked, 'Why were you not Moses?' Instead, I shall be asked, 'Why were you not Zusya?'" Shakespeare wrote: "To thine own self be true. Thou canst not then be false to any man." And, Richard Bach in *Illusions* echoed the sentiment: "Your only obligation in any lifetime is to be true to yourself. Being true to anyone else or anything else is the work of a false messiah."

I will be forever grateful for my experiences at the ashram. I said my goodbyes with the usual mixed emotions. "J'ai bhagwan. J'ai bhagwan." I felt whole, cleansed, loved and loving. I also felt ready to return home, to my family, to the outside world; I was ready to integrate all my new awareness into my life.

A New, Healthful Reality

One of the first things I did when I got home was to open our "important papers" box and pull out my birth certificate. Sure enough, it verified that my biological parents were the parents I had always lived with and that I did, indeed, belong to my family. I was NOT found on the doorstep in a basket. This was now clear in my mind once and for all. It is remarkable to consider how deeply our beliefs affect us. I couldn't help laughing at myself for checking my birth certificate immediately upon my return, despite all the profound realizations I had just processed at the ashram.

Could there be any doubt that what we believe becomes our reality, whether it is true or not? If I believed that I had been abandoned, left on a doorstep in a basket, making me unworthy of love and attention, how could I ever possibly believe I was good and lovable? I got the message in the depth of my being that I did not deserve love simply because I existed; I had to earn it. I had to work hard for love, always being there for others, especially for the family who took me in. I had to be perfect and to be helpful always because therein lay my value.

Interesting that the unconscious fear I had of rejection and abandonment attracted a mate who would perpetuate my feeling of not ever being emotionally safe. That must have been life's way of giving me a present situation that would trigger unresolved past issues so that I could confront them and resolve them. To live more fully in the present, I had to complete the past. I knew that I came down with MS for many sound reasons. The disease was a manifestation of my breaking of some important universal laws.

I was beginning to understand what disease is all about. Our bodies are the barometers of how we are doing with all that we put into them, including all the mental stuff that we experience. If we are doing okay, processing and applying what we're learning here on earth, our bodies feel pretty good. We have a good energy level. We're sleeping well. We're eating well, and our body systems are carrying out their work without too much stress and strain.

One of the most common symptoms in most diseases is fatigue. Coincidentally, one of the most common symptoms of people who deny or repress their true selves and honest feelings is also fatigue. Such people are not so much tired as they are tired of. Their sense of loss of muscular power is more of a sense of loss of soul power, or loss of control over their own lives. I can now appreciate the vast effort and energy it took for me to hide behind a smile so often and to deny rather than acknowledge my true feelings.

I had been following through with what I accepted from my early messages; never before had I questioned why I felt that my very existence depended upon how good a caretaker I was. I just kept trying harder and harder to be all things to all people, until the cumulative stress from this overwhelming effort, together with the enormous energy it took to repress and deny my own needs, burst through in a disease called multiple sclerosis. Then I was forced to take an inner look and to understand who I really am, where I've been and where I was headed. MS forced me to find ways to let all the negative messages of the past go and to be at one with myself again.

I also had to practice letting go in my current life and to learn what that meant. I discovered that to let go meant getting rid of my compulsion to help, my need to fix it for others. It did not mean to stop caring; rather, it meant admitting that I can't do it for someone else. To let go meant not to care FOR but to care ABOUT. It meant not to fix but to be supportive, not to protect but to permit another person to face reality. I learned that to let go is not to deny but to accept. It is not to enable but to allow learning from natural consequences. To let go is not to try to change or blame others; it is to make the most of myself.

When I let go of my past, I did not regret what had happened to me; rather I appreciated the opportunity for growth, understanding and completion. I learned to fear less and love more, to trust my intuition, to trust the process of life. Most of all, I learned to keep in constant touch with that deepest place within, the place that never changes, the place that is non-judgmental and filled with unconditional love, pure love and acceptance for myself and all others.

Most of us were subjected to early negative programming. This programming is often the very basis for the way we create our own reality. We experience life based on what we accepted and believed about ourselves and our environment when we were very young and impressionable.

The good news is that it is always possible to reprogram ourselves. With conscious effort and conscious choices, we can remove the effects of those early negative messages. Once I discovered where my need to be needed came from and how I was carrying on old habits in current relationships, I could begin to grow and change. I realized that my desire to fix it for my husband was self-destructive. I would never be able to help him put the ordinary obstacles of life into some kind of perspective. I would never be able to help him feel some kind of *joie de vivre*. My compulsion to help him kept me from fulfilling my own needs. I neglected myself, abandoned myself and left my spirit bereft. I created the perfect conditions for a disease to move in and thrive.

Once I realized that it was not within my power to fix it for my husband, I also came to the awareness that I could still be supportive of him. I can respect his right to be who he is. I can accept him as he is, with the full knowledge and understanding that he has every right to be exactly who he is. On the other hand, I can no longer permit him or anyone else to violate me. *I have every right to be who I am. I don't have to be perfect; it's much more important to be perfectly me.*

After my second visit to the ashram, I told my children the full story of my struggle to recover. I named the disease that the doctors had diagnosed. I gave my children all the details then because by that time I knew that I was going to get completely well. I had enough confidence in my own hope to deal with any doubts they might have. I knew that I was improving and that my improvement was not a remission. I knew that if I kept in touch with my own lovely spirit, I could work wonders. I continued to look long and hard into my inner mirror. I no longer ignored or repressed my real feelings; there was no need to. I was coming from a more realistic and honest base. I was more connected to who I really was. It was incredible to feel that I was one with myself again.

My goals and my life were changing dramatically. I experienced many moments of private personal growth — insights would appear suddenly, fade and then reey finally became integrated into my

hildren had all graduated from college
ng on their own. My husband was con-
s routine. Our marriage was more utilitar-
y thing else. My need was to concentrate on
mpletely well. I combined all I had learned
y childhood messages with the changes in diet
and the therapies I had previously implemented. This
holistic approach seemed to be working. The process
was slow and excruciatingly tedious. But gradually I
got rid of the walker and then the cane. I was able to
walk securely on my own again. I had normal strength
in my arms and hands and in my legs and feet. My
balance and energy level were restored. I no longer
suffered from overwhelming fatigue.

Although I had the feeling and control back in my
right leg and foot, I still was not walking as smoothly
and evenly as I once had. This might have been from
overcompensating to balance myself for so long. I had
no idea what the reason for my jerky walk was, but I
was concerned about it. Just as I had been guided so
often earlier, once again a teacher did appear. It came in
the form of a statement that I remembered reading. I
must have been ready for it. It appeared in my consciousness and seemed to take on important new
meaning. I grabbed a pen and wrote the words on my
shopping list:

> *The me I see is the me I'll be.*
> *If I cannot see it, I will never be it.*
> *Until I believe it, I will never achieve it.*

I had never heard of imagery or visualization. Those
concepts did not have widespread popularity in 1977,
the year I began practicing my own invented version.

When I remembered the rhyme, I immediately tried to act as it was advising. I focused on the words, centered myself and tried to see myself walking properly.

I kept at this for several weeks, even trying to get into a more meditative state for seeing myself with a smooth, even walk. But I didn't seem to be making any progress. I thought maybe the technique wasn't working because I could not see myself in very much detail, and I could not focus clearly.

Once again, I knew of no authorities who could guide me. I decided to thumb through magazines until I found a picture of a woman walking with a nice stride. A photograph of the actress Barbara Eden caught my eye. She was walking purposefully and gracefully across the page. I tore her photograph out of the magazine. Then I found a snapshot of myself and cut my face out of it. I pasted my face onto Barbara Eden's body.

Before going to sleep each night and upon arising each morning, I would deep breathe myself into a relaxed, meditative state and I would focus on that picture. I found that I was able to hold the image of my face on Barbara Eden's body clearly and in great detail. I kept the image in my mind until I could actually see myself in full stride and walking gracefully. This exercise twice a day did wonders. Before too long, I noticed an improvement in my walk. It really worked for me.

The visualization of actions appears to help train the brain to send appropriate neurological messages to the muscles involved. Today there are many books about imagery and visualization. There are also workshops and courses for anyone who wishes to explore this phenomenon. Your local community college, library or health food store can help you get started.

Twelve years after being diagnosed with MS, I was completely free of any symptoms. In fact, I felt better than I had ever felt in my life. The journey back to health had been an amazing one for me. The recuperative power of my body will never cease to astonish me. Once I was healthy again, I began getting back into the mainstream. I started seeing old friends more often and making new ones. I pursued my many interests. Through word-of-mouth, many people learned of my recovery and sought my advice for health problems of their own. The tremendous interest in the path that I followed was one of the reasons I decided to write this book.

Several of my friends had divorced after their kids were grown and gone. It was becoming more common for couples to take stock and realize at that time in their lives they were growing away from each other, going in different directions. Their expectations for the remainder of their lives were dissimilar, and the consequences were irreconcilable.

Just as my husband had not involved himself in my long struggle back to health, he was unable to share in my healing and liberation. I did hear from others about how proud he was of my successful effort to recover. I accepted him simply as he was and honored his right to remain that way. I was supportive of him without making any effort that would help us grow together. The distance between us became increasingly wider. Eventually, and before I had lost all symptoms of MS, we were divorced. It was an amicable parting. He, as well as all of us are products of our past with multi-generational programming running through our veins. MS motivated me to confront mine in order to put a halt to my self-defeating choices.

This story is not about blame. There are no right or wrong answers . . . there are only questions and individual choices. There is never a need to blame when we can understand and appreciate why we need to attract a particular manifestation in our lives. I thank my ex-husband for his many fine qualities. I thank him for the good, kind, loving person within that he had to mask at times. I thank him for the whole experience that was yesterday. My fondest wish for him is that he find a way to understand his own self-defeating behavior. I wish that he could understand, appreciate and let go of his guilt. I wish that he could give himself permission to be the good, kind, loving person that he is masking within. Most of all, I wish him a better relationship with himself; that is where all good things begin.

My entire experience of recovery was undeniable. Many people ask how I can be sure that my disease is not just in remission, even though I have been free of symptoms for more than ten years now. Multiple sclerosis is characterized by a come-and-go pattern. Symptoms usually appear and disappear without warning. The appearance of symptoms is known as an exacerbation; the disappearance, as a remission. Both exacerbations and remissions are spontaneous in nature; the person with MS suddenly develops a new symptom, or an existing symptom suddenly goes away. My recovery was nothing like a remission. There was nothing spontaneous about it. It was excruciatingly slow

and painstaking. First I gained back so
I had lost. Then I built up some stre'
and toes. My progress was so grad
observe it from one day to the ne'
all of my time for twelve years.

There is much scientific evidence ധ.
the techniques that I used to heal myself. I believe, as
do countless others who have also recovered from so-
called incurable diseases, that the significant factors
involved in my recovery were:

1. The imperative inner journey, where I found
   answers that allowed me to reshape my innermost self.
2. Persistence in the struggle for health.

I will repeat that my health returned after a long,
excruciatingly slow and difficult struggle. It was not a
gift; I earned it. Most people are not willing to take the
kind of time that I took to reclaim my well-being. My
recovery certainly was not a spontaneous remission. It
was the result of hard work and a stubborn insistence
on the question, *Who said so?*

As I was working my way back toward health, the
process became as important — if not more important
— than the goal. Indeed, the process and the goal
seemed to merge until they became the same thing. The
process of my journey to recovery has given me the
kind of resourcefulness that will see me through any
event in my life. If I had a crisis every hour, I know I
could deal with it. This is an incredibly powerful feeling.

All Answers Are Within

*Power comes to those who know they
know.*

— *Karl Menninger*

Throughout my search for health and
growth, my intuition played a primary role. Since the
medical community paradoxically fostered dependence
yet could offer me no help, I did not have much else to
go on. Why not play my hunches?

What I wanted most, in the beginning, was some
authority to guide me. I could not get what I wanted.
But I did get what I needed. I needed to learn that I
could trust my inner feelings, my inner knowledge, my
instincts and intuition. I needed to acknowledge that I
carry the answers I seek within myself. The life process
demands that we go within to find our lasting answers.
Discovering the need to do this may take a lifetime. I
call this dipping into the divine knowledge, which is
our link to the universe. We never betray ourselves
more than when we do not follow our innermost
knowing. Trusting the knowledge that comes from
within is crucial to any healing. Ultimate healing is our
own enlightenment.

I wanted to understand more about our intuitive
nature, so I read everything I could on the subject. I

learned that the intuitive mind, unlike the rational mind, has an organic quality. The intuitive mind thinks with images and feelings and, by necessity, works in harmony with the whole being. If we have been out of touch with our real feelings, our inner selves, we lose sight of how powerfully useful the intuitive mind can be.

The tools that are most useful in unlocking mental powers, or bringing the intuitive mind to consciousness, are meditation, visualization and journal keeping. Keeping a journal, which is not a diary but more like a place for brainstorming or writing down everything that comes to mind, takes us back to our intuitive nature by clearing the mind of its busy-ness.

The more we awaken our intuitive nature, the more we are able to grasp our life in a holistic way. When we follow what our intuition tells us, we have more energy because we are headed in our own natural right direction. This is what usually turns us on and makes us more creative, effective and powerful. Intuitive knowing is a higher form of knowing than rational knowing. Rational knowing limits us to fact, whereas intuitive knowing can also encompass truth. Intuition can be weakened by conventional education. But it can be strengthened by conscious, deliberate effort. The choice is up to us.

Space travel and scientific data have given us a clearer perspective on the cosmic forces that continually flow through us. Each cell in our bodies is a vital link with the order that governs the universe. Intuition is our link to our inner selves and our higher consciousness.

Now all health communities believe that our mental, emotional and spiritual states of being cannot be separated from our physical well-being. All systems are interconnected. There is constant communication between body and mind. Illness in the body reflects disharmony on all levels. When there is physical dysfunction, the message is to examine all areas of our being — our thoughts, attitudes, beliefs and feelings. The need is to examine what is not working in our lives, to discover what our true needs are and how to get them met. We must restore the natural harmony and peace between our inner and outer selves.

There is divinity in each one of us. We are divine expressions of the principle of creation on this level of existence. Our connection to the universe is our higher self. It speaks to us through instinct and intuition. We can call this higher self by many names, including inner self, divine self, intuition, spiritual nature, inner voice, soul, love nature, heart nature, higher consciousness, instinct, inner guidance, essence, very core, true self, real self, God self. All are one and the same. This self remains constant, no matter what is happening in an ever-changing, chaotic world. This higher self is the place where my busy mind, my overwrought emotions and my fatigued body come home for strength, hope and serenity. This is the bottomless filling station, the nurturing place, the place of renewal, the place of boundless love, of divine wisdom and knowledge. This is the common meeting ground for me and the outside world. Here my inner wisdom and my outer self merge to become one in guiding me toward choices that are in my best interest. Here is the source of my strength to endure, to integrate what I learn and to make contact with universal energy and love, which is boundless and forever available. Here is my place to rest and renew, to process and prioritize.

Perfectly Me and Perfectly You

The way to do is to be.
— *Laotzu*

The alienation that we all feel at times is primarily in our minds; we have tuned out that necessary intuitive heart place. I know how often I neglected my inner self in my frantic attempts to be perfect, to fit in, to fix it, to achieve, to be accepted and to become. How much more sense it makes simply to be.

Good health demands that we keep in touch with, value and constantly acknowledge that intuitive heart quality which introduces us to the love of ourselves and others. When we can get back in tune with it, our lives are more peaceful meaningful, loving and lovable. Our hearts resonate one to another.

Even after we secure all the things we think we want (family, job, home, money, car, etc.), there is still an emptiness. This void has driven many a high-powered executive to return to a simpler life. Mother Teresa calls this void "spiritual deprivation." There is a growing recognition that spiritual poverty may be more devastating than economic poverty.

There was a time when I thought a spiritual person was someone in a white robe, meditating on a Himalayan mountaintop. I now know that spiritual people are very much like you and me. They are all around us, trying to overcome and correct their own weaknesses while being tolerant of everyone else's shortcomings. Spiritual people are those of us who have the strength to be vulnerable and show our loving selves to the world. We have known non-judgmental awareness and unconditional love, and we want to share those glorious feelings.

Recently, I read a "Stress Awareness Questionnaire." I found that I had enough of the stress factors in my life to be a candidate for a major illness. However, I was in good health. The stressful events were not affecting me physically. I was getting a divorce, adjusting to the empty nest, toughing it out on my own on considerably less income than I was used to, moving out of the home I had lived in for twenty-five years, living alone for the first time in my life, living in a small apartment in an unfamiliar city, having no family or friends nearby. Shortly after I moved, I fell in love. The relationship was nearly perfect for two years. Then he died suddenly of a heart attack, leaving me with an unbearable loss that I will feel forever. As one more stressful event in my life, I undertook the monumental task of writing my very first book.

Any two of these stressful situations would have made me a likely candidate for an exacerbation of the MS or for another major health crisis. Yet, I continued to improve. Although my recovery has been put to many a test, I have experienced no illness, no symptoms, no exacerbations, nothing, not even a headache.

In *The Healing Heart*, Norman Cousins wrote that just before he had his first heart attack, he knew he was stressed and overtired. He tried to get out of some of his commitments. His secretary said that there was nothing on his itinerary that she could cancel. She added, "It's not as though you had a heart attack or something."

When she said that, Cousins's body was listening. Cousins, one of the most influential figures in uncovering the mind-body connection, definitely believed in a direct link between what goes into the mind and what happens to the body.

According to Arnold Hutschnecker, author of *The Will to Live*, if you feel trapped in a situation, if you can't logically work out your priorities and attitudes to deal with that situation, your body will give you the excuse you need. If you are lucky, you will get away with a minor illness.

When we have a need to justify ourselves in the eyes of others, we are setting ourselves up for stress and the resulting emotional or physical illness. Many people have to give up the self-indulgence of trying to be considered right in order to become well. The reality is that no one is perfect. You don't have to be perfect. Everyone is better served if you are just perfectly you.

Being Independently Healthy

It's no matter to die. But it's a terrible thing not to live.
— *Victor Hugo*

My own experience taught me that disease is not just a matter of invading germs or viruses or a degenerative process, but that the reason for any illness can be traced to the way a person is living. We can be set up for disease by self-defeating behavior that is programmed into us when we are very young. Until we confront and challenge these early messages that we receive from our families, we will continue to be victimized by them. We will be stressed and negative, and our spirits will be bereft. Our immune and central nervous systems will suffer.

There is now much evidence to support how and why I recovered from MS. The recommended reading list in the back of this book lists the authors whom I have found most persuasive and illuminating on the topic of healing and wholeness. I came from a place that said I had no alternatives to a place that said the choice was mine. The medical community, at the time I was diagnosed with MS, fostered dependence but offered neither help nor hope. I had to go outside the system in many different, unrelated directions to search, to experiment and to make a career out of trusting my own instincts and intuitive nature. In other words, I was forced to become my own authority.

My journey from acupuncture to Adelle Davis to Dr. Evers to Shangri-La to the ashram to my inner self was all under my own direction. It was a journey into uncharted territory. It was a risk that I had to take. I had no forerunners, no authority figures, no guides until I finally realized that the best, purest and most powerful guidance possible was available to me — my very own unique intuitive nature was there to lead me in the right direction. I needed to let go of the pressures and turn off my rational mind in order to find the answers. Healing is an inside job.

Our innermost knowing will always reveal what is uniquely right for each of us if we take the time to make a conscious effort to keep in touch with that all-knowing, inner part of ourselves. By getting into a relaxed state and dipping into the divine knowledge, we can always find the next step to take. I searched and investigated relentlessly until I accomplished what I had set out to do. I was not addicted to results or guarantees. I knew only that I had to go forward using whatever I could find, learning from every situation, remaining open, trusting my intuition and following through with whatever made sense to me.

The reinforcement that I got from my very first step out on my own — the experience with acupuncture — gave me the courage and the drive to continue on my own. From this, I learned that regeneration is possible, even though I had been told that there was no cure for MS and I should not spend my energy looking for one. Each subsequent risk that I took brought more positive reinforcement. As I saw myself improving, I was able to tune out the negatives I encountered and derive sustenance from the increasing number of positives.

When I was first told that I had an incurable, life-threatening disease, what I wanted most was some medical help and guidance. I DID NOT GET WHAT I WANTED. BUT I DID GET WHAT I NEEDED.

I learned that the specifics of HOW TO need not be understood first. Once we have a deep conviction and make a genuine commitment for change, the mind-body connection will get the message at the cellular level. We will intuitively gravitate toward finding out all the specifics of HOW TO. Most of us try to work this process in reverse. We frantically involve the will and the mind, trying to learn all the facts that we can, gathering all the evidence. We try so hard, and we waste a great deal of energy. When we can actively involve our inner selves (our all-knowing, intuitive, spiritual nature), we become more connected and influenced holistically. We don't have to figure out how to; the specifics will present themselves to us.

Our early programming has conditioned most of us to fear and limitation. We need to have a more realistic perspective on our own possibilities and potential. We need to integrate self-belief and self-acceptance into our daily lives so that positive change is inevitable. We humans are magnificent, recuperative miracles and natural overcomers. We create our own reality with our perceptions, thoughts and beliefs. One of the most important things I learned is how to begin again. But first I had to let go and let things come to their natural ends.

Through my search, I learned that health and healing are best approached on several different levels: physiological, psychological and spiritual. The name of the disease does not matter. Illness strikes when the body is not functioning properly; resistance is low and the immune system is not defending as intended. When the disease attacks, it goes after the weakest part of the person.

On the physiological level, I took the approach that I wanted to cleanse my body and avoid chemicals. I learned about natural hygiene, a detoxification and elimination program. I dropped all meat from my diet and changed to primarily raw, live foods, eaten in the proper combinations. Enzymes that are found mostly in raw foods are important in digestion. Many health problems and degenerative diseases are a result of the lack of these enzymes. I learned that our bodies are composed of individual cells that are constantly wearing out and being replaced by new cells. The new cells are built from the material in our food. Nature affords us the remarkable ability to rebuild ourselves day by day from the food we eat. Rebuilding cells with live, uncooked foods gives our systems less work and helps our immune system function better. Outside viruses and germs have trouble taking hold in a body that is naturally regenerating itself. When we eat the proper foods, we give our bodies the materials they need to enhance their own recuperative powers.

I also learned the importance of exercise and body movement. I kept everything moving that I could and added parts as their mobility was restored.

On the psychological level, I learned the importance of dealing with stress and pressure in a direct and constructive manner. Healing happens when we de-congest the mind and emotions of early programming and negative thoughts, replacing them with self-love and life-affirming behaviors and choices. It is not the original childhood trauma itself that causes the problems we live with; rather, it is the repression of the trauma or the negative messages that we believe about the trauma. There is no pain comparable to the pain of trying to avoid pain. After all of my years of trying to repress or cover up my hurt and pain over one theme of my childhood, I have to conclude that the more we push the feelings away, the more we push ourselves away. And the worse our pain gets. The grief work — feeling those sad, awful wounds all over again, dredging them up in order to understand them — is necessary if we are to break the hold of those wounds on our lives.

If anger is one of the emotions that you have suppressed, you must find a way to release it. Most people tend to suppress anger. They keep it so deeply buried that they aren't even aware of having any anger. This tendency is developed early in life. The blocking of such a powerful emotion will take its toll on the body. One good anger-releasing technique is to pound on a mattress with a tennis racquet. If you are generally shy and afraid of violence, this will help you find your inherent strength and assertiveness. You won't have to be afraid any more. You will know that you are strong and can respond with anger when it is called for. This exercise is a compromise between inhibiting genuine emotions and doing yourself or someone else actual physical damage. If you allow yourself the regular release of pent-up anger through this safe exercise, you will be doing yourself a vital service.

This is the technique: Kneel on a pillow beside your bed. If you like, imagine someone there at whom you feel angry. It could be someone from your current life or someone from your past. It could be your boss, parent, sibling, spouse, child, employee, etc. Raise the racquet up over your head, and as you bring it down, say, "Take that" or even say words you might usually keep yourself from saying, such as, "I hate you" or "Leave me alone." Repeating "No No No" as you pound the racquet on the bed is also an effective way to release your frustration and rage.

This tennis racquet technique is a method recommended in Lisette Scholl's *Visionetics*, an excellent book that is, unfortunately, out of print. Scholl cautions that you might not get instantly in touch with your anger as you hit the mattress. Your defenses might take over and try to immobilize you by making you feel weak, hopeless or anxious. If this happens, she says, and your breathing becomes tight and you feel depressed and dizzy, just sit there and breathe deeply and slowly into those feelings. Accept the feelings and reflect on what this defense against anger might mean to you and your body.

Everyone needs to find a constructive way to rid the body of trapped anger. If you don't want to try pounding a mattress, how about screaming in the woods? Or writing all your angry feelings in a letter to whoever is making you feel that way? Don't send the letter; tear it up.

I shudder to think of where I would be had I ignored my instinctual and intuitive nature. If I had accepted my doctor's prognosis as all-knowing and final, I would have undoubtedly declined exactly the way he predicted. Had I chosen to believe that MS was incurable, I would have made no effort to help myself find ways to get back to the good, healthy, radiant life I am enjoying today. If we accept a prognosis without question and seek no further on our own, we can indeed make the prognosis come true.

The spiritual level of recovery may be the most important. Nothing can substitute for the search in our souls for beauty and love. Good health begins with the inner journey back to loving ourselves.

I don't know why so many of us find loving ourselves so difficult. One of the best ways to begin is by never criticizing ourselves for anything. When we criticize ourselves, we are usually saying, "I am not good enough." We criticize ourselves because we have bought into the messages from our early programming. Those messages made us feel, as children, that we were not good enough. When we grew up, we continued to believe that we were not good enough. Until we leave these childhood perceptions behind, we are powerless to be present. We cannot learn who we really are.

Self-acceptance and self-approval are crucial to good health and positive change. Progress happens when we can love and approve of ourselves just as we are, even with the qualities that we used to think of as not good enough.

When we understand and appreciate that all healing begins within, we will work at letting go of fear, of blame, of self-criticism, of the need to judge ourselves and, therefore, others. When we drop all the negatives, we are unmasked. What is left is our very essence, which is love. Only love remains. We are just the way we were born — pure love. When we come from a place of love, we spontaneously view others with love. We see their higher selves rather than their hurting selves. We see their essence instead of their negative, love-starved behavior. Healing happens when we accept ourselves and others as unique and perfect manifestations of this pure-infancy-essence, love.

It is not my intention in this book to persuade anyone to accept what has been proven true for me. This is my reality. Your reality will take some involvement on your part. The involvement alone can open up your life in a unique and promising way. I respect anyone's right to remain in the status quo. But I also passionately encourage those who want to feel what life has to offer beyond the limitations of disease and circumstance. I believe we all have a timetable and we are exactly where we are meant to be at a given time. You can learn a great deal from others who have gone before you in this kind of work, but you do not have to depend on them. Trust yourself. And always question, "Who said so?" Always ask, "Why?" Bear in mind the advice given to the cub reporter: "Trust your mother, but check it out for yourself." The biggest truth is that all the facts are never in.

If you could travel the distance that I and many others like me have traveled to get where we are today, you would have no doubts about your own ability to accomplish anything. You have the tools — you have instinct, logic and common sense. You need commitment and an attitude that understands we are not victims of the world we see; rather, we are victims of how we see the world. The very quality of your life depends on your attitude. Your attitude toward yourself affects your attitude toward others and toward every area of your life.

Consider the person who is wearing a fifty-pound stone around her neck. As long as she thinks of it as a stone, her attitude is that it is intolerably heavy and nothing but a burden. But notice how her attitude changes when she learns that it is a precious stone, a diamond. Her load is suddenly lighter. She welcomes it. The weight of the stone did not change. Only the person's perception of the worth of that weight changed.

What could possibly be more important than your perception and your attitude? Together, they create your reality, the very world in which you live. Attitude is always a choice. If you want to know what your tomorrow will be like, simply examine your attitude today.

Consider the case of the bumblebee. All the wisdom of human science says that the bumblebee should not be able to fly. That fat body and those short wings — poor aerodynamic design; it should never get off the ground. The bumblebee, however, has not had its attitude infected by the wisdom of human science. It goes right on flying because it knows it can.

For true seekers, there is always a way. I am living proof of this. In a degenerative disease, it is the patient, rather than the doctor, who makes the difference. If we participate in our health care instead of acting like hopeless victims, we can significantly aid in our healing as we increase the quality of our lives. Feelings are chemical. You cannot fool your body. Your emotional condition influences your immune system. If you deny your needs long enough and do not respond emotionally, your body will speak up for you.

Disease can actually result from a lack of unconditional self-love. The underlying reality for all human beings is that our very essence is love. Love is our connection, our source of energy, our divinity. We come into this world as an entity of love. I learned to begin self-love by discontinuing any self-criticism and by appreciating all my good qualities. I learned to support my real moment-to-moment needs as an act of self-love. I gave myself time for relaxation, contemplation and meditation, all of which helped me reinforce my inner knowing. We are empowered when we recognize and acknowledge that we know.

My intuition told me that some kind of growth was going on inside me. All disease is rooted in a spiritual crisis that manifests in the body in order to get our attention. My spiritual crisis came about because of neglected needs, my neglected inner self.

If overcoming disease leads you to trust your own intuition, you can think of your disease in a very positive way. Healing yourself can be the most valuable time in your life. I now know that I am my most authentic authority. I was privileged to have experienced that unbeatable combination of the spiritual and the practical.

My hope is to leave you with a million questions, starting with, "Who said so?" I cannot supply your answers. Ultimate healing is your own enlightenment. You are your own best authority.

Appendix

Studies of the effects of stress, which can be caused by physical tensions like exhaustion or by psychological strains like grief or anger, show that the mind is as involved in sickness and health as the body. Today, a new understanding of how body and mind interact is evolving, one that takes into account the relationship between stress and other emotional responses and the onset development and outcome of illness. Remind yourself frequently that health and healing come from within, not in any mystical sense, but by means of real physical connections. The way you think and feel influences those connections. If your mind now hinders them, you can train it to help.

— *Dr. Andrew Weil in* Health and Healing: Understanding Conventional and Alternative Medicine

Health-Enhancing Techniques

The following pages describe briefly some of the alternative healing methods that I explored.

Mini-tramp

I started using this small trampoline shortly after I began my water exercises in the pool. Because of my weakness and poor balance, I was not able to stand and jump on the mini-tramp. I could, however, sit on it and bounce up and down. I decided to do this after reading that the jumping motion increases cardiovascular efficiency, improves lymphatic circulation, increases energy and allows you to get the maximum amount of exercise with the minimum amount of effort. If you cannot sit on the mini-tramp, you can sit in a wheelchair next to it and put your feet on it while someone else jumps. This enables your body to experience some movement.

Shiatsu

Also known as acupressure, reflexology or zone therapy, this healing tradition from the Far East dates back thousands of years. It is the practice of applying finger pressure to penetrate the pressure points along the energy pathway meridians. Practitioners learn to project chi, or the life force, through the hands, transferring it to the patient to unblock the stagnation that has led to pain, stress and disease.

Rolfing

This technique of deep body massage was developed by Dr. Ida Rolf, who believes that gravity puts considerable stress on the human body, which must consequently be realigned. In Rolfing, the practitioner brings the major segments of the body—head, shoulders, thorax, pelvis and legs—toward vertical alignment. Rolfers prepare the body to receive and respond positively to the effects of the gravitational field.

With any physical ailment there is mind and emotion involvement. Rolfing accentuates the mind/body connection by removing the physical blockages that inhibit the flow of information from the mind to the body through neurotransmitters.

Chelation Therapy

The purpose of chelation is to remove the calcium deposits from the intimae of the blood vessels. Chelation does improve circulation throughout the body, and the increased circulation helps to supply added nutrients to the nerve fibers. Theoretically, then, chelation could aid in the re-myelination of the nerve fibers.

Chelation therapy is being performed in this country by nutritionally oriented physicians. It is a somewhat controversial therapy. Dr. Hans Neiper reports success in Germany and Sweden with an oral chelation used to treat MS patients. My own experience with chelation was inconclusive; I cannot say whether the treatments improved my condition.

Diet

I first learned about the benefits of eating raw fruits and vegetables when I was at the Shangri-La Natural Hygiene Institute in Bonita Springs, Florida. What I discovered there was reinforced when I went to the Hippocrates Health Institute, which was opened in California in 1976 by Raychel Solomon. Nothing is ever cooked at Hippocrates. In fact, there is no stove in the kitchen. The meals are all uncooked vegetables, fruit, seeds and sprouts, in amazing variety. I learned about the importance of raw food and food combining, and I took classes in digestion, elimination and detoxification of body and mind. The classes were taught by Patricia Wing, a registered nurse who had overcome a life-threatening cancer through the nutritional approach outlined in the Hippocrates program, and with the therapeutic use of wheat grass.

The original Hippocrates Health Institute, on Exeter Street in Boston, was founded more than thirty-five years ago by Ann Wigmore, who is a pioneer in living foods research. There are numerous documented cases of healing as a result of Dr. Wigmore's teaching, and they involve every disease imaginable.

It is with deep gratitude that I recall my many visits with Raychel Solomon and Hippocrates West, which is now called the Health Institute of San Diego and is located in Lemon Grove, California. The incredible foresight, conviction, fortitude and inner strength of this caring, beautiful lady has brought meaningful education, health and healing to the many thousands who have participated in her programs. Once again I was privileged to experience that unbeatable combination of the spiritual (nature's best) and the practical that makes it all possible.

Keep starches and proteins separate.

In my study of natural hygiene, I learned that it is best not to combine proteins and starches in the same meal. Starches begin to digest in the mouth and proteins in the stomach. This means that when the starches begin to break down and go to the stomach, they encounter hydrochloric acid, which has been released there to digest the protein. The starches then begin to ferment, causing indigestion, flatulence and discomfort.

Correct Food Combining
Monotrophic Meal—One Food at a Meal is the Ideal.

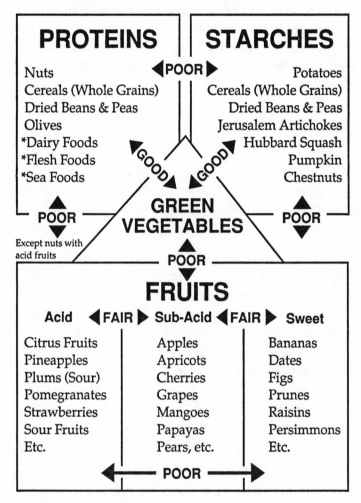

Avocado — Combines well with all foods except proteins and melons.

Tomatoes — may be taken with non-starchy vegetables and protein.

Melons — Eat them alone or leave them alone.

* These substances not recommended but included for clarity.

© Copyright by The Shangri-La Natural Hygiene Institute, Bonita Springs, Florida 33923-PA

Avoid hydrogenated fats.

Hydrogenated fats are found in foods like cookies, crackers, cakes, candy, potato chips and granola. Hydrogenated means that the fats have hardened and will clog the arteries. You should also avoid palm, cottonseed and coconut oils, all of which have high hydrogenated fat content.

Eat garlic to cure whatever ails you.

Garlic is reputed to be a powerful detoxifier, nature's antibiotic as well as nature's tranquilizer. Paavo Airola in *The Miracle of Garlic,* writes:

> *Garlic, the miracle healer, in controlled and reliable clinical studies, has shown to improve conditions such as: high blood pressure, athersclerosis, tuberculosis, diabetes, arthritis, cancer, hypoglycemia, bronchitis, asthma, whooping cough, pneumonia, common cold, allergies, intestinal worms, intestinal putrefaction and gas, parasitic diarrhea, dysentery, insomnia, coagulation disorders, upset stomach, grippe, sciatica, chronic colitis, gastritis, emphysema, athlete's foot, worms, constipation, intestinal disorders, colds . . . .*

J.D. Knofsky M.D., in an article entitled "A Pungent Proposal," reviewed the abundant literature on garlic and came to the conclusion that we might all have much better health if we ate a bit more garlic. Kanofsky found that garlic lowered blood pressure, blood cholesterol and triglyceride levels; inhibited the clumping of blood cells that sometimes precipitates strokes; and decreased the risk of hardening arteries.

I use garlic medicinally, particularly for colds and to lower my blood pressure.

Take papaya for indigestion.

The fruit papaya is full of natural enzymes that counteract stomach acidity. Most health food stores carry a product known as papaya enzymes, which is very effective when taken after meals.

Don't forget your chicken soup.

The Mayo Clinic has finally given its blessing to a remedy that Grandma has always known about—homemade chicken soup. The soup seems to play a part in clearing up the respiratory system. It could be tried before any drugstore cold remedies.

Eat more fiber and less fat.

Keeping the colon clean is imperative. A clean and normal colon makes a large contribution to happiness and well-being. An abused colon leads to the spread of poisons throughout the body. Fiber helps keep the colon functioning properly by soaking up water from the intestine as it passes through. The fiber then becomes bulky and moves down the bowel more quickly. It encourages faster movement through the colon, thereby helping rid the bowel of wastes and toxins in less time.

Fat, when it comes into contact with the normal bacteria found in the bowel, makes a chemical that scientists think may cause cancer. Also, the body has to produce certain acids to digest the fat (bile acids); scientists think these may also produce cancer. The consensus is that a high-fiber, low-fat diet can reduce the incidence of cancer of the bowel by at least thirty-five percent.

Breath as a Tranquilizer

If you are having trouble getting to sleep, try slow breathing from the diaphragm. Breath, which is nature's tranquilizer, can work wonders.

First Aid for Sprains

Packing the injured area in a few slices of lemon brings quick relief from sprains. The citric acid seems to draw out the heat and swelling and also promotes healing.

Dental Considerations

Some multiple sclerosis patients reportedly have experienced some symptom reversals after having the silver fillings removed from their teeth and replaced with a non-metal composite.

Improved Circulation

Soak your feet for about twenty minutes in warm water to which you have added about six ounces of grated ginger. You will notice an improvement in circulation. Also great for circulation is to roll your bare arches (one at a time) back and forth over a Coke bottle on the floor. Or, you can purchase a wooden device called a "tootsie roller" at a health food store.

Stretching to Begin the Day

You insult your body when you hop out of bed without stretching in the morning. I recommend stretching from head to toe while you're still in bed and then doing a few knee-to-chest pulls. This initial stretching will increase blood circulation and ease muscle stiffness. You will arise with a happy body. Take a lesson from what the cat does upon awakening.

Drug-free Pain Remedy

There are many pain clinics that do not use drugs to relieve pain; they use relaxation techniques. Giving a suggestion to each part of the body to relax is much healthier than risking the toxic side-effects of drugs. Imagery and visualization are also being used successfully for pain relief. They are powerful tools for physical, emotional and mental health and well-being.

Relief for Burns

Good first aid for burns is to pierce a vitamin E capsule and put the contents on the burn. Or you can squeeze the gel from an aloe vera leaf onto the burned area.

Stronger Stomach and Abdominal Muscles

The best exercise for strengthening the muscles of the stomach and abdomen is simply to hold the stomach in constantly, without holding the breath. Visualize a long zipper being pulled up from the pubic bone to the waist. Zip it up as often as you can.

The Necessity of Perspiration

Perspiration is one of the ways we eliminate waste and toxins from our bodies. It is most important to our health. Yet we are bombarded with advertising messages that tell us perspiration is something of which we should be ashamed. Do not become hypnotized by these unsafe messages. And be sure when you purchase any deodorant that it does not stop the flow of perspiration, as an antiperspirant is meant to do.

Some researchers believe that there is a link between the use of antiperspirants and breast cancer. When we clog up the poisons in our bodies by using antiperspirants and when we subject our bodies to the aluminum compounds that antiperspirants contain, we are causing ourselves real problems. The body absolutely needs to perspire. Odiferous perspiration comes chiefly from internal toxicity, i.e., when there is putrefaction inside the body from food that has not been digested properly.

Laughing Matters

> *God is a comedian, playing to an audience*
> *that is afraid to laugh.*
> — *Voltaire*

Laughter is contagious. If you are lucky enough to catch it, pass it along.

Illness is not a laughing matter, but perhaps it should be. Laughter is a form of internal jogging. It enhances respiration and is an igniter of great expectations. Nothing can aid in relaxing the tension in the body like laughter.

No longer considered frivolous, play and laughter are acknowledged to be important in making friends, releasing the stress of daily life, combating illness, promoting better self-image and better relationships in business and enhancing communication, productivity, cooperation, creativity and camaraderie. A sense of humor reduces the importance of the ego and puts life in perspective. A sense of humor also recognizes the universality of life. When people laugh together, it is because they share a common value system. Comedy unites people. It can be a wonderful relief and a great leveler for the human condition. Comedy is about living in this world just as it is. When the chaotic world gets to us and we are helpless to change it, we can poke fun at it and maintain our health and sanity.

"Research shows that humor aids most — and probably all — of the major systems of the body," says Dr. William F. Fry, a psychiatrist at the Stanford University School of Medicine and author of three books on humor and health. He adds:

A good laugh gives the heart muscles a good workout; improves circulation; fills the lungs with oxygen-rich air; clears the respiratory passages; stimulates alertness hormones, which stimulate various tissues; alters the brain, diminishing tension in the central nervous system; counteracts fear, anger and depression, all negative emotions linked to physical illness; relieves pain.

Humor is all over, if you look for it. It doesn't take any effort to put more smileage in your life. Humor brings instant relief from unbearable pressure. Laughter makes the body function much more efficiently. Laughter also changes body chemistry in a very positive way. If you laugh a lot, when you get older, your wrinkles will all be in the right places.

Why take life so seriously? You'll never get out of it alive.

Humor makes life worth living. Life is a celebration. Make it fun for yourself and others.

The Twelve Pathways

One of the lecturers and writers most helpful to me in this aspect of my personal growth was Ken Keyes. I believe that his Twelve Pathways are essential knowledge for all who would restore their spirits. Keyes' pathways are a variation on the ubiquitous and extremely useful twelve-step program developed in Alcoholics Anonymous. The person who doesn't have an addiction and would not go into a twelve-step program can benefit greatly from following Keyes's twelve pathways, which I am reprinting here with his blessing:

THE TWELVE PATHWAYS

*To the Higher Consciousness Planes of Unconditional
Love and Oneness*

Freeing Myself

1. I am freeing myself from security, sensation, and power addictions that make me try to forcefully control situations in my life, destroying my serenity and keep me from loving myself and others.

2. I am discovering how my consciousness-dominating addictions create my illusory version of the

changing world of people and situations around me.

3. I welcome the opportunity (even if painful) that my minute-to-minute experience offers me to become aware of the addictions I must reprogram to be liberated from my robot-like emotional patterns.

Being Here Now

4. I always remember that I have everything I need to enjoy my here and now — unless I am letting my consciousness be dominated by demands and expectations based on the dead past or the imagined future.

5. I take full responsibility here and now for everything I experience, for it is my own programming that creates my actions and also influences the reactions of people around me.

6. I accept myself completely here and now and consciously experience everything I feel, think, say, and do (including my emotion-backed addictions) as a necessary part of my growth into higher consciousness.

Interacting With Others

7. I open myself genuinely to all people by being willing to fully communicate my deepest feelings, since hiding in any degree keeps me stuck in my illusion of separateness from other people.

8. I feel with loving compassion the problems of others without getting caught up emotionally in their predicaments that are offering them messages they need for their growth.

9. I act freely when I am tuned in, centered, and loving, but if possible I avoid acting when I am emotionally upset and depriving myself of the wisdom that flows from love and expanded consciousness.

Discovering My Conscious-awareness

10. I am continually calming the restless scanning of my rational mind in order to perceive the finer energies that enable me to unitively merge with everything around me.

11. I am constantly aware of which of the Seven Centers of Consciousness I am using, and I feel my energy, perceptiveness, love and inner peace growing as I open all of the Centers of Consciousness.

12. I am perceiving everyone, including myself, as an awakening being who is here to claim his or her birthright to the higher consciousness planes of unconditional love and oneness.

Rainy Day Box

When times were darkest for me, when I despaired of ever making any progress, when I wondered why I was going against the entire medical establishment, I could always find some comfort or reassurance in what I called my Rainy Day Box. This was an old cigar box, which I had covered in a scrap of wallpaper. Into the box, I put any encouraging words I could find: quotes that seemed particularly meaningful to me (many of them are included in this book), cards from friends and family who wanted to express their feelings of love and affection for me, accolades I had received from my various volunteer efforts in the community. My Rainy Day Box affirmed my self-worth and the worth of my struggle toward health and wholeness.

A Happy Little Ditty

I feel that the following little ditty helped me counteract some of the negative messages from my limited childhood perceptions that may have lodged in my cells, influencing my health and behavior. The little ditty was given to me by the Reverend Pierre Gallardo of Las Cruces, New Mexico. This was a constant; if I was not softly singing it to myself, it was rolling around in my head — always:

> *I deserve to be healthy.*
> *I deserve to be wealthy.*
> *I deserve to be happy and strong.*
> *With each breath that I take,*
> *All my cells rejuvenate.*
> *And I love to affirm this song.*

Recommended Reading

Bradshaw, John. *Healing the Shame That Binds You*. Deerfield Beach, Florida: Health Communications, 1988.

Chopra, Deepak. *Quantum Healing*. New York: Bantam Books, 1989.

Cousins, Norman. *The Healing Heart*. New York: Norton, 1983.

Davis, Adelle. *Let's Get Well*. New York: Harcourt Brace, 1965

De Vries, Arnold. *Therapeutic Fasting*. Green, Iowa: Chândler Book Company, 1963.

Hutschnecker, Arnold. *The Will to Live*. New York: Crowell, 1951.

Remen, Naomi, *The Human Patient*. Garden City, New York: Anchor, 1980.

Samuels, Mike. *The Well Body Book*. New York: Random House, 1973.

Siegel, Bernie. *Love, Medicine and Miracles*. New York: Harper & Row, 1986.

Weil, Andrew. *Health and Healing: Understanding Conventional and Alternative Medicine*. New York: Houghton Mifflin, 1983.

Other Books You May Find Useful...

☐ *Gentle Yoga* by Lorna Bell, R.N. and Eudora Seyfer
This book is especially designed for people with arthritis, stroke damage, or multiple sclerosis, those in wheelchairs, or anyone who needs a gentle, practical way to improve their health through exercise. Includes over 135 helpful illustrations.
$9.95 paper or $12.95 spiral, 144 pages

☐ *How Shall I Live?* by Richard Moss, M.D.
A medical doctor and alternative healthcare advocate discusses how to deal with a major health crisis, and how to transform the experience into an opportunity for greater aliveness. Covers issues such as fear, guilt, helplessness, and despair and shows how to release and share your healing energies.
$8.95 paper, 180 pages

☐ *Staying Healthy with Nutrition* by Elson Haas, M.D.
The long-awaited examination of how what we eat determines our health and wellbeing. Truly a complete reference work, it details every aspect of nutrition, from drinking water to medicinal foods to the latest biochemical research.
$24.95 paper, 1,168 pages

☐ *Wellness Workbook* by John Travis, M.D. and Regina Ryan
An updated edition of one of the first books on total wellness–how to integrate physical, emotional, intellectual, and spiritual factors to create vibrant, life-long health.
$13.95 paper, 256 pages / A TEN SPEED PRESS BOOK

☐ *Healing Environments* by Carol Venolia
This holistic approach to "indoor well-being" examines healing, awareness, and empowerment, and how they are affected by various aspects of our environment. Its principles can be applied to homes, workplaces, and healthcare centers to bring greater peace and harmony into our lives.
$9.95 paper, 240 pages

Available from your local bookstore, or order direct from the publisher. Please include $2.50 shipping & handling for the first book, and 50 cents for each additional book. California residents include local sales tax. Write for our free complete catalog of over 400 books and tapes.

Ship to: Celestial Arts

Name_____   P.O. Box 7327

Address_____   Berkeley, CA 94707

City_____ State ____ Zip _____   For VISA or Mastercard orders

Phone _____   call (510) 845-8414

                                                              (800) 841-BOOK

"While many valuable books have described successful fights back from heart disease and cancer, *Who Said So?* by Rachelle Breslow is one of the first books to recount a victory over multiple sclerosis. People facing MS will benefit from her experience and her dogged faith in her own intuition and healing power."

— *New Age Journal*

"This book is written extremely well and stands out from the vast sea of self-help books. It will both touch you and inspire you. Any person facing serious illness (including AIDS) would benefit from Breslow's story."

— *The Unicorn*

"I found myself fascinated with Breslow's experience and read *Who Said So?* within two days. I found that its messages apply to us all, whether or not we are experiencing any illnesses or dis-ease. Her healing is an inspiration for all as we look within to rediscover our true power and perfect health."

— *Mighty Natural Magazine*